EMBODIED BEING

Also by Jeffrey Maitland

Spacious Body

Spinal Manipulation Made Simple

Mind Body Zen

EMBODIED BEING

The Philosophical Roots of Manual Therapy

JEFFREY MAITLAND, PhD

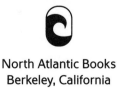

North Atlantic Books
Berkeley, California

Published by
North Atlantic Books
Berkeley, California

Cover art by Volterrano (Baldassare Francheschini), *Truth Illuminating Human Blindness*, about 1650. Digital image courtesy of the Getty's Open Content Program.
Cover design by Jasmine Hromjak
Book design by Brad Greene
Printed in the United States of America

Embodied Being: The Philosophical Roots of Manual Therapy is sponsored and published by the Society for the Study of Native Arts and Sciences (dba North Atlantic Books), an educational nonprofit based in Berkeley, California, that collaborates with partners to develop cross-cultural perspectives, nurture holistic views of art, science, the humanities, and healing, and seed personal and global transformation by publishing work on the relationship of body, spirit, and nature.

North Atlantic Books' publications are available through most bookstores. For further information, visit our website at www.northatlanticbooks.com or call 800-733-3000.

MEDICAL DISCLAIMER: The following information is intended for general information purposes only. Individuals should always see their health care provider before administering any suggestions made in this book. Any application of the material set forth in the following pages is at the reader's discretion and is his or her sole responsibility.

Library of Congress Cataloging-in-Publication Data
Names: Maitland, Jeffrey, 1943–
Title: Embodied being : the philosophical roots of manual therapy / Jeffrey Maitland, PhD.
Description: Berkeley, California : North Atlantic Books, [2015] | Includes bibliographical references and index.
Identifiers: LCCN 2015035427 | ISBN 9781623170264 (paperback)
Subjects: LCSH: Manipulation (Therapeutics) | BISAC: HEALTH & FITNESS / Massage & Reflexotherapy. | HEALTH & FITNESS / Alternative Therapies.
Classification: LCC RM724 .M32 2016 | DDC 615.8/2—dc23
LC record available at http://lccn.loc.gov/2015035427

1 2 3 4 5 6 7 8 9 UNITED 21 20 19 18 17 16
Printed on recycled paper

~ for Lee-Ann ~

CONTENTS

Surprised I Still Had Toes

My professional education as a psychiatrist taught me observation, knowledge, and thinking. Our patients had bodies, of course. Yet it was their minds we focused on. Personal experience plus over three decades of psychiatric practice taught me just how vital *embodiment* is to all aspects of health. I know we must pay attention to bodies, at least as much as to minds.

Embodied Being is about coming home to our bodies and to our authentic selves. From here, we become free to love and live and flourish at our best. On the other hand, a chronic lack of being fully embodied appears to be a source of chronic and sometimes severe suffering. I have found that this suffering is rarely relieved by the mind's thoughts or by talking therapy alone. Holistic somatic/manual therapists can be essential to the homecoming process.

I know personally the importance of being at home in my body. I began to learn this thirty years ago when my daughters died. Almost immediately, I became numb. I no longer could feel my body or my emotions. I looked down and was surprised I still had toes. I clearly still had a body but could not feel it.

It has been a long journey back to being embodied. In trauma, our bodies are wired to help us survive by moving painful memory and emotion out of our awareness. We do not intend for it to happen. It just does. It is part of the built-in way we protect ourselves. Disconnecting from feelings and pain in this way was life-saving for me, at the time. Eventually, I felt a strong urge to reconnect, come home to my body. Finding my way back meant, among other things, retrieving those feelings and memories that were out of awareness. I learned these were stored not in my mind (or what some might call the subconscious) but deep in my body, in the soma.

Dr. Maitland argues that there is no such thing as the subconscious. I agree! So did neuroscientist Candace Pert, PhD, who said, "The body is the mind's subconscious." When our minds or nervous systems become overwhelmed and unable to process what is happening, it is the body with its observable energy field that astonishingly holds for us those important feelings and memories for safekeeping until it is time to release and harvest them for their healing potential.

The body's brilliance appears in how it defends against releasing these at an unsafe time or in ineffective order. I have had the experience of working with therapists who were skilled therapists, good people. My body opened to their intention and skill, but then it quickly closed down even harder because it was not the right timing or order of release for my particular issues. It was crucial to find somatic therapists who can "see" holistically in ways that helped me release, in a safe way, what was stored.

This book's brilliance is found in something rare in books on manual therapy: a richly tempered philosophical approach coupled with new and practical methods for learning to "see" holistically through all the senses, including a sixth sense. The book elegantly lays out a newly created three-step self teaching process in how to "see" holistically. The book also states the principles of intervention, perhaps for the first time for some manual therapists, and shows how to use them to good effect. The complicated process of designing treatment strategies is boiled down to answering three simple questions: What do I do first, what do I do next, and when am I finished?

As a trained philosopher, Rolfing instructor, and Zen monk, Dr. Maitland travels far in this book—from the breadth and depth of philosophy's elegant language and arguments to down-to-earth plain-speak that often surprised me with words that quickly turned complexity into what is simple and relevant.

One such phrase I particularly like is "order-thwarters." Basically, when all is well, bodies and minds have an innate rhythm, smooth flow and natural order. When flow is interrupted, the natural order is thwarted. Order-thwarters can have many faces. They may be myofascial restrictions, distortions, and complicated strain patterns throughout the body from birth trauma, trauma at any age, falls and accidents, illness, low back pain, exhaustion, joint fixations, fear, pain, faulty worldview, war, addictions, threats and dangers from outside, untimely deaths and losses, natural disasters and much more. Order-thwarters can be sensed by sensitive, holistic, somatic therapists who know how to "see" and properly apply and dose his or her remedies. Dr. Maitland's sections on how to identify and approach order-thwarters are to be savored.

In this book, Dr. Maitland often discusses philosopher René Descartes. I see Descartes as someone for whom natural order appears to have been thwarted from the start of his life. From birth, his mother was unavailable to him due to her illness and subsequent death by the time he was a year old. With nurturance, infants gradually learn to embody, touch their toes, smile at others and view the world. Sadly, Descartes did not have this in his early life. He apparently did not experience embodied being.

In my opinion, Descartes's lack of being at home in his own body seems part and parcel to his often quoted line, "I think, therefore I am." Without the nurturance adequate to become embodied, being in his head to think was all there was. "I think, therefore I am" seems to me to be very sad. I hear it as a statement of existence, but not of heart or authenticity or truly vibrant am-ness. Yet, his words have become so ingrained in our language and belief system as to almost antidote the reality of body and its importance.

I know from experience of this separation of mind from body. Fortunately, before my daughters died, I had some experience of being in my body. Afterward, when I could not feel my toes or my body, I couldn't feel emotions either. They, too, were numbed. It felt as if my body was cement; I just could not get in there to feel. It was uncomfortable. I no longer had "gut reactions." I could not tell if I wanted tea or coffee. I no longer knew how to make decisions. The best I could do was to try to figure it out with my mind. And that was not easy or, frankly, very successful. It led to mistakes. But, I remembered what being in my body was like and longed to be there.

I am grateful to the wise, holistic somatic therapists like Dr. Maitland who helped me to return home and to the smooth flow of natural order. I hope his new and stunning book, *Embodied Being*, will be read by many therapists, and by people whose ways of coping by thinking and intellectualization have worked to some extent *and* who now want to explore further, if only a tiny bit further, into embodied being.

JUDITH S. FREILICH, MD
OCTOBER, 2015

INTRODUCTION

This book is not a manual of techniques. My previous book, *Spinal Manipulation Made Simple*, is a clear example of such a book, but it—unavoidably and like other manuals of its type—cannot give us a way to prioritize all the information we have gathered from our assessments into a coherent and effective treatment strategy that sequences interventions in the appropriate order. In short, a manual of techniques tells us where to work, but not when or in what order. Skilled manual therapists have been creating effective treatment strategies for so long that they no longer give much thought to how they do it. If they are called upon to say what they are doing, they often rightly emphasize the importance of assessment at the beginning, during, and after performing therapy. But characteristically they have trouble finding words to describe a remarkably accurate and uncanny perception of patterns of fixation and dysfunction (to capture their inherently relational nature, I call dysfunction and illness "order-thwarters" and will expand on this term in Chapter Two). Since remarkable perceptual skills are so poorly understood and so difficult to talk about, exploring how to *see* gets lost in almost every attempt to lay bare the clinical decision-making process. It is not too surprising that all such attempts often leave us struggling with a vague sense that something important is missing.

Many experienced practitioners exhibit an uncanny ability to see/feel into and through the body's order-thwarters both locally and globally and at the same time. They are capable of tracking both the release of local order-thwarters and the effect on the body as a whole as it reorganizes itself. Their perceptual prowess often educes flummoxed amazement from novices as well as a deluge of questions such as, "Why did you work here instead of there?" or "How did you see that?" or "How did you know there was a connection between the adductor attachments of the left leg and the base of the occiput?" Not understanding the source of such uncanny perceptual skills any better than the novice who wants to learn them, the experienced practitioner sometimes feels inadequate over a loss for words and replies in frustration, "Can't you just see it?" This answer is about as helpful as blaming the whole thing on intuition. Typically, this kind of discourse leaves the hapless beginning practitioner with no idea of how to go about seeing what the experienced practitioner saw.

When it comes to manual therapy, skilled perception is at the heart of every assessment and central to the practice. But be careful not to limit the use of the words "perception" or "seeing" to the visual alone. As you read further into this book, you will discover that we are able to perceive with more than our senses. If you cannot see what is troubling your client, you are not ready to perform manual therapy. Skilled perception and being able to perform a thorough assessment are essential to the therapeutic process. But how do we train practitioners to cease being bystanders who have narrowed their assessments to only looking for joint restrictions, finding "tight" myofascia, or listing symptoms instead of *seeing* what the body wants to show them? It is fairly straightforward and easy to objectively measure range of motion, time a client when walking from point A to point B, or simply point out that a client's head is too far forward, or that his or her legs are too valgus. But where, for example, does the ability to see a pattern of angry energetic/fascial strain connecting with a person's low back pain come from? How do we become uncanny seers, or, more to the point, how do we stop looking and begin *seeing*?

These considerations are acutely relevant to the practice of holistic manual therapy where seeing the wholeness of the client is crucial. Seeing holistically is much more difficult and all-encompassing than piecemeal assessments. It is a way of seeing that is most akin to aesthetic appreciation, where you have to see the whole all at once in the details and become more expansive and go deeper while participating in the very act of seeing itself. You have to give up your stance as an onlooker/bystander in order to let what is show itself to you. You also have to be prepared to see all manners of phenomena that cannot be simply categorized as subjective or objective. You must learn to trust your senses, cultivate your perceptual acuity and vitality, and remain open and receptive to whatever shows itself.

Most practitioners would probably agree that holistic seeing is one of the most important skills a practitioner can develop. Given how important perception is to manual therapy, it is surprising how little attention is paid to understanding and cultivating it. Unfortunately, it is barely understood, and finding a workshop devoted to cultivating skillful perception is next to impossible.

Once I realized what was missing from the resources, I set about trying to create a self-teaching training exercise. The result is a simple three-step exercise based upon insights I gained from years of practicing Zen, Rolfing Structural Integration (Rolfing SI), philosophy, and phenomenology. But, by far and away, the most potent insight came from Goethe and the way of seeing he called "exact sensorial imagination." At last, I had found a way to train students in the art of seeing. Because of his subtle and refined perceptual abilities, I enlisted the help of Advanced Rolfing Instructor, Ray McCall, and we collaborated and taught a workshop on *seeing*. The philosophical background for this exercise is found in Chapter Six, and the exercise itself appears in Chapter Seven.

Besides the theory and practice of perception, there is one more critical piece that has been missing in most attempts to understand the clinical decision-making process—a working knowledge of the principles of intervention. Important as it is, perception alone is not sufficient for showing you how to sequence your interventions. It might not be an exaggeration to say that the most popular word in the literature of manual therapy is "principle." But nowhere do you find any indication of what meaning of "principle" is being used. On top of that, what most theorists list as principles of intervention are, in fact, not principles of intervention at all. Chapters Three and Four are designed to remedy this situation.

To bring this discussion into sharper focus we can pose three fundamental questions that face every therapist whether you are a shaman or a surgeon: what do I do first, what do I do next, and when am I finished? To answer these questions you need to be skillful at applying techniques, you need to be able to perform thorough assessments, you need to be trained in how to perceive, and you need to know the principles of intervention and how to apply them in the therapeutic setting. This book is designed to show you how to meet these four needs.

The meaning of the word "rational" is very suggestive. It means to think in accordance with principles. In an effort to free Rolfing SI of formulistic protocols and create a rational principle-centered decision-making process in its place, Senior Advanced Rolfing Instructor Jan Sultan and I developed the principles of intervention while teaching an advanced Rolfing class together. Michael Salveson, also a Senior Advanced Rolfing Instructor, added some needed refinements later. Part of this book is about delineating the details of what we developed and how to put it to good use.

My training is that of a Rolfer. As you might expect, Rolfing comes up for discussion here and there. Many of the examples I cite are of people who have received Rolfing. As you read you will see, however, it is a book about manual therapy, not a book about Rolfing. Manual therapy is a comprehensive inquiry into the theory and practice of caring for and enhancing our embodied uprightness. Rolfing is just one of many comprehensive manual therapy disciplines. I am not interested in trying to say what the essence of Rolfing is in order to show how it is uniquely different from all things not Rolfing. In the end, there is nothing unique about being unique. The power lies in what is common. Accordingly, this book is about the kinds of philosophical and practical issues that face every Rolfer, therapist, manual therapist, and health care provider. These issues are universal. They are not limited to Rolfing or manual therapy alone.

When Western philosophy got around to grappling with the mind-body problem, much more attention was given to deconstructing the mind than the body. Instead, I reverse the order of investigation and begin with the body. Nevertheless, my approach is not just the cerebral, conceptual approach of a philosopher to the body instead of the mind. Rather, I begin with the body as it discloses itself subjectively when it is in the process of receiving manual therapy. Having been a professor of philosophy, I am quite familiar with and have great respect for the queen of the sciences. While it is true that philosophy informs my approach to these matters, years of Zen practice in exploring the "end of the mind road" has made me equally wary of its limitations. As a result, I have learned to pay attention to how the subjectivity of the client's body whispers its needs to the therapist's subjectivity. Since I have devoted many years to exploring how to listen to these whisperings, it is highly probable that this very practical, hands-on approach informs the content and style of this book more profoundly than the conceptual/philosophical approach.

This book is also written loosely in a style of thinking the Chinese call round thinking. It is a way of thinking that discloses the nature of holistic phenomena. To engage in round thinking is to think and perceive holistically. Since holism is at the core of manual therapy and biological order, it is discussed at length. Because of the way holistic thinking continually circles its subject matter, deepening understanding by adding new information as it goes, it sometimes appears overly repetitious. But, in the holistically organized sentient body, all roads lead to wholeness. The repetition characteristic of round thinking is in the service of deepening and expanding understanding.

Whether we fully realize it or not, how we practice and understand our version of manual therapy often rests upon unexamined philosophical presuppositions that breed confusion. One of the most important influences on how we see the world comes from the philosophy of René Descartes and the theory that has come to be called metaphysical dualism (see especially Chapters One and Six for a discussion on this theory). His influence on how we see the world is both pervasive and perverse—so much so that many of us accept a view of reality that is at odds with the kind of *seeing* that is at the heart of holistic manual therapy. Because they cannot be easily characterized as objective, skillful holistic assessments are viewed with suspicion, and often considered a form of idiosyncratic subjectivity.

This book could rightly be seen as a study in the meta-theory of manual therapy. But, first and foremost, it must be seen as a philosophical work, informed by philosophy throughout. It brushes up against such lofty topics as the previously mentioned metaphysical dualism, the nature of perception, the nature of human freedom, embodiment, and the quest for our true home. It also offers a possible first step in the solution to the age-old mind-body conundrum. Along the way, we also take excursions into how holistic manual therapy can open us to the numinous. Most of these existential concerns transcend the usual practical issues that face manual therapists in their day-to-day activities. But when these more existential concerns surface for a client, manual therapy reveals valuable insight into what it means to be a happy person at peace with him- or herself and the world. Because manual therapy has much to teach us about ourselves, these existential concerns are tightly woven into the text and approached in terms of how we experience them, that is, in terms of how the experience feels to us. As a result, this book also should be of interest to those who do not practice manual therapy, but are interested in what a science of subjectivity looks like when it is practiced as manual therapy.

I wrote this book to make room for the kind of reality and perception Descartes's philosophy could never recognize or appreciate. I followed a line of thought that at first felt like catching a loose thread. As I pulled on it, I felt the Cartesian worldview begin to unravel. At the end of the thread I discovered the sentient (self-sensing) body uncovered first by Maurice Merleau-Ponty. In time I realized that what I was calling "the sentient body" was a clear example of consciousness as a somatic event. As a result, consciousness and body were no longer two mutually exclusive incommensurable ontological types. The discovery of the sentient body (or reflexive flesh) is a critical step in toppling the hegemony of the Cartesian worldview. The importance of the sentient body to this study is taken up in Chapter Eight.

There is more to do, but enough unraveling has occurred to justify setting the Cartesian worldview aside. And as a result, we can rest assured that our holistic assessments and ways of *seeing*, even if they do not fit easily into the framework of subject and object, are every bit as veridical as what our senses reveal.

Where Descartes was in search of certainty of knowing, I found myself more interested in pursuing the certainty of being—in cultivating the clear-minded imperturbability so characteristic of coming home to our bodies. At this level of understanding, the practice of manual therapy can become a laboratory in which you pre-reflectively explore what is true and possible for our lives, beyond but not in opposition to the confines of subject/object distinction. For the client, continued manual therapy can serve to enrich the experience of embodiment and further the evolution of self-development and freedom.

CHAPTER 1

Homecoming, Part 1

Of all the things that inhabit this vast universe, nothing is more enigmatic than what is closest to us—our own nature. We know ourselves to be conscious beings, capable of both abstract thought and complicated emotions. But as soon as we try to say what consciousness is or how it exists, we quickly find ourselves embroiled in a morass of philosophical confusion. Things are not much different in our attempts to understand our emotions. But perhaps the most elusive of all is our own embodiment. The more we try to grasp it, the more easily it slips away.

We are embodied beings. What could be more obvious? Whether we experience great sorrow or irresistible joy, it is our body that undergoes the experience. It is not enough to say you understand a joke if your body is not moved to laughter. Getting a joke is laughing at a joke. Similarly, if you are listening to a piece of music and you are not moved by it, you probably are not appreciating it. From the deepest samadhi ever imagined to the most cerebral experience ever conceived, the body always participates. To talk about experience is already to talk about the body.

Yet, a cursory look at the history of Western philosophy reveals an astonishing lack of nuanced attention to our bodily being. Instead of an examination of what it means to be embodied, we find no shortage of disparaging remarks about the body. The body is often seen as a nuisance always getting in the way of our more intellectual/spiritual concerns. As Nietzsche observed, "Were it not for the fact that man has a gut, he would think of himself as a God." Given that all experience is bodily, it is most surprising that no sustained philosophical understanding of our somatic nature appears until the twentieth century. This kind of historical legacy should give us pause and remind us to hold our presuppositions up for careful examination throughout our investigation.

The roots of our understanding of the body go back some 2,500 years ago to the dawn of Western philosophy when Plato put forward the view that mind and body are separate entities. Known as metaphysical dualism, Aristotle famously captured Plato's position when he said that the mind is to the body as the pilot is to the ship. Because Plato recommended that we fastidiously care for our bodies, he was clearly no hair-shirted ascetic. But he was not exactly a fan of our embodiment either. He considered the body a lesser reality than the mind and claimed that the body was the prison house and the disfigurement of the soul. Centuries later, Galileo and Descartes added to metaphysical dualism the idea that the body is a soft machine, prompting twentieth-century philosopher Gilbert Ryle's clever remark that in Descartes's view a human being is a "ghost in a machine." As we shall see, even though metaphysical dualism has received a great deal of critical attention, some of its most problematic assumptions still inform our view of the body and hence how therapy is delivered and received by the client. From the beginning to the end of our investigation of manual therapy, we will, therefore, continually not only call into question the pervasive problematic assumptions associated with metaphysical dualism, but also suggest possible ways to refurbish some of our key concepts. We will also lay out the principles of intervention and a three-step method for training those perceptual skills that are necessary and essential to assessing clients within a holistic approach to manual therapy.

From Symptom to Self-Discovery

When clients seek the services of a manual therapist, they are typically looking for improvement in their functionality. They may want relief from their aches and pains or better coordinated possibilities of movement. Once these goals are achieved, satisfied clients terminate their therapy. Though free of their pain, some clients are not changed in any fundamental way. In contrast, other clients are so dramatically changed by their therapy that their life takes a surprising new direction. Clearly, their therapy was not just about treating their symptoms, curing their disease, or getting rid of back pain. It was also about something more existentially comprehensive and compelling. It was also about completing the self, about maturing and becoming who they truly are. And in finding themselves they also discover where they belong. "To touch" also means "to ignite," and it is clear that the touch-based therapy they received ignited in them the age-old quest for self-knowledge and illumination.

These dramatic differences in results are due to radically different approaches to therapy. A great many practitioners attempt to alleviate the client's problems by treating symptoms in a piecemeal way. As we shall see, it is significant that these practitioners tend to be metaphysical dualists who believe the body is a soft machine. In contrast, the holistic practitioner tries to bring harmony, order, and balance to the whole of the client. In the case of Rolfing, one further requirement is added—to facilitate the integration of the body and the environment in gravity.

Both approaches can relieve the client's aches and pains, but the holistic approach can become more like an education in completing the self— how to become who we are—rather than an exercise in simply easing symptoms. Symptoms are not ignored or considered unimportant in the holistic approach. Symptoms are addressed along the way, but are not seen as isolated events. Symptoms are understood to be modifications of larger patterns. The main event is not symptoms, but the lack of integrated balance in gravity and the effect larger patterns of strain have on the body as a whole. The holistic approach is good at relieving pain, facilitating functional economy, and normal coordinated movement. But the holistic approach also has the potential to accelerate the completion of the mature self. By speeding up the maturation process, clients are put more in touch with themselves. As they appropriate more and more of their freedom, they more and more experience the joy of finding themselves and their place in the world.

If you are not familiar with the holistic form of manual therapy, you may be surprised to learn that such an approach is capable of such global change. In fact, there are quite a number of holistic therapies capable of such far-reaching changes. The holistic approach is capable of creating new possibilities for the future by erasing the patterns that bind us to a dysfunctional past. It can so profoundly reshape the body that there is no longer any room for emotional torment. It can free you of pain. It can release your joy and put you in touch with the true nature of things. It can teach you how to move with grace. It can open your heart and introduce you to the numinous.

Of course, not everyone who undergoes the holistic approach will get the same results. The experience of harmony, order, and integrated balance to which holistic therapy aspires can be shallow or deep. Many people are simply not prepared for or interested in pursuing the heights to which holistic therapy sometimes ascends. Many just want relief from their pain. But for those who are ready, it can be a liberating experience. A good way to capture this experience is to see it through the metaphor of homecoming.

Waking Up to Your Feeling-Nature

The Buddha is reported to have said, "The foot feels the foot when it feels the ground." With this statement he clearly recognized the reflexive character of consciousness. Unlike a mechanical apparatus, when a living creature senses something, it also senses itself sensing. No matter how rudimentary or complex something is, if it is capable of reflexivity (self-sensing), it is possessed of sentience. Sentience is common to all living creatures. With respect to human consciousness, we can say that human consciousness arises as a wildly complex elaboration of sentience coupled with the evolution of language. We will return to the idea of sentience and the discovery of the sentient body in Chapter Eight.

We live in an ocean of sentience. But because our consciousness is dominated by the stance of an onlooker who narrowly objectifies reality, we no longer trust the information we can gather by means of feeling. We are thinking creatures. But we are also feeling creatures possessed of a remarkable ability to perceive by means of feeling. Practice the three-step exercise in holistic seeing described in Chapter Seven, and you will discover this ability for yourself. Continue to practice the three-step exercise and you will discover that you can perceive with your whole body. You will come to see from your own experience that thinking and feeling are two deliquescently related aspects of the sentient whole that is your body.

There is no word for this ability to know or perceive by means of feeling. I refer to it as our feeling-nature. Perhaps you have had the experience of accurately feeling that something is amiss just before entering a room. Another common experience is the feeling of being watched and turning around to discover someone staring at you. These examples are just two among many possible experiences of your feeling-nature at work. Your feeling-nature can function as an organ of perception that lives in every nook and cranny of your body. It is not just limited to particular emotions or feelings alone. Your very ability to feel this or that particular emotion or feeling depends upon having a feeling-nature in the first place.

The more we practice clearing ourselves of our order-thwarters, the more we can trust what our feeling-nature shows us. To be able to rely upon it and use it in the practice of manual therapy we must exercise it. Eventually, the clear-minded imperturbability characteristic of embodied freedom will be part of how we approach every session. I will return to a more detailed discussion of our feeling-nature in Chapter Five.

The metaphor of homecoming is well-suited for describing the potential of the holistic approach. At this point in our exposition, it will be more useful to appreciate the aesthetic aspects of self-discovery before we delineate the important details of how holistic manual therapy is practiced and differs from the more common approaches. To that end, we will examine the metaphor of homecoming as a way to get a felt-sense of what the results of holistic therapy look like to an observer and feel like to the client. This process of letting the potential of holistic manual therapy show itself through the metaphor of homecoming will assist us in getting to recognize and appreciate our feeling-nature and its manner of perception. It will also help to guard us against prematurely succumbing to empty abstractions in the place of felt-lived experience.*

If you can imagine how it feels to live your body in a fluid, light, balanced way, free of pain, stiffness, and chronic stress, imperturbably clear minded, at ease with yourself and with the gravitational field and environment, then you will have some sense of what it means to be embodied and you will understand part of what a holistic approach like Rolfing can achieve. The experience of coming home is an adventure in self-discovery. With it comes joy and a deep sense of gratification that results from being in agreement with your circumstances, finding your self, and feeling like you belong. Suddenly, the world feels like a great work of art. It seems to exhibit an astonishing level of habitable orderliness and connectedness that is difficult to express in words, but is perfectly obvious to the whole of your feeling-nature. This kind of order is not driven by OCD or any neurotic need for neatness. In the grand simultaneity of things, the harmony we feel with nature, a beautiful piece of music, or in homecoming is the same. We feel at ease in a world that seems designed to bring us pleasure in just being here enjoying the freedom of embodiment.

Following Samuel Todes's lead we recognize that we are creatures with a need for a habitable world.[1] As we all know, the world is not always an easy place. It is filled with many difficulties and obstacles, small and calamitous, man-made and natural, which frustrate our attempt to make our way. We find ourselves inexplicably thrown here in the midst of circumstances where the way is not always clear. It can leave us feeling lost, alienated, or lacking a sense of belonging. At the same time, things are not always all bad. Coming into agreement with our world and gratifying our need for habitable order brings with it varying degrees of freedom and ease. We cannot change the fact that everything changes, nor can we rid the world of all its dangers and obstacles to our path. When we come to finally understand that freedom is the creative appropriation of limitation, we discover how we can and do find

---

*For more on the perceptual capacities of our feeling-nature, see my book *Mind Body Zen* (Berkeley: North Atlantic Books, 2010).

ways to make our world habitable. And the most profound way to make the world humanly habitable is to free our feeling-nature and body of conflicts and fixation. Such a body can more easily adapt to changing and difficult situations. It can, as we say, "roll with the punches."

"The world of human experience is the humanly habitable world, not just because we make it so, but because the world enables us to make it so."[2] We are able to be at home and at ease in a world that makes sense to us because the world appears designed to provide us with the means to make it so. We know from evolutionary biology that the organism and its environment evolve together. A relationship in which organism and environment evolve together would provide an organism with a powerful evolutionary advantage. It is certainly reasonable to assume that ours is just such a favorable enabling environment.

The Need for Order

A surprising place in which to find a way to describe coming home is in the aesthetics of Immanuel Kant (1734–1804). Although Kant does not make this comparison specifically, because of the close connection between beauty, order, and feeling-based judgments, a case can be made that his analysis of the appreciation of beauty can also serve as an elucidation of the experience of homecoming.[*]

For Kant, the appreciation of beauty is not a frivolous pursuit of pleasant experiences. The power of beauty to profoundly move us lies in its ability to engage us in the free play of the same cognitive processes we employ in the pursuit of knowledge. As cognitive beings we are always in search of knowledge. In advance of any experience of order, we are prepared and ready to find order. But, because we are also limited beings, we can neither fully comprehend nor prove this order. Therefore, in order

---

[*]For a more in-depth approach to Kant's aesthetics than I can provide here, see my article, "An Ontology of Appreciation: Kant's Aesthetics and the Problem of Metaphysics," *Journal of the British Society for Phenomenology* 13, no. 1 (January 1982): 45–68.

to practice science we must adopt a heuristic principle that assumes that nature is in harmony with our rational demands for order.

In the appreciation of beauty, this heuristic principle is unexpectedly confirmed and we find ourselves at ease and at home in a humanly habitable world filled with beauty. The appreciation of beauty gives us an experience similar to the profound gratification we feel when we make breakthroughs in our pursuit of knowledge. We are profoundly moved in the appreciation of beauty because it sets in motion the same harmonious, orderly, intellectual activity that we enjoy when we are engaged in research. In the appreciation of beauty, however, we are freed from the constraints and rigors of the kind of rationality required by the pursuit of objective scientific knowledge. As a result, we can revel in the joy of coming home to a world that appears specifically designed and ordered for us. The pleasure we feel is the product of the deep gratification that comes from experiencing that our need for order is profoundly confirmed. Although there is no designer, natural beauty seems specifically designed to give us the kind of pleasure we as cognitive beings would most enjoy. The important difference between science and the appreciation of beauty is that beauty comes into being without the benefit of concepts. Ultimately, beauty is the non-conceptual revelation of the activity through which all of this appears and disappears. Great works of art and the beauty of nature are windows to the world before it is conceptualized.

You do not have to agree with all the details of Kant's approach to appreciate the depth of understanding involved in describing what it feels like to come home. It is significant that both Todes and Kant see in us a deep need for orderliness. Remarkable as Kant's elucidation is, however, something critical is missing. Conspicuously absent from Kant's exposition of the kind of orderliness revealed in the appreciation of beauty is any reference to the body. Surely, the delight and ease we feel in the presence of beauty is also a bodily comprehension. Great art and the beauty of nature *move* us, sometimes profoundly. They do not just give us a pleasure limited to cerebral free play. Our feeling-nature is joyfully released in the vertical. Being embodied means that we have found our true home, and our whole body participates in the appreciation of beauty and the experience of self-discovery it calls forth. This kind of joyful homecoming is nothing if it is not comprehended by our feeling-nature and body as a whole.

Beauty

Kant's aesthetics allowed us to uncover this deep-seated need for order at the heart of our quest for knowledge. But this constitutive need is not limited to our cognitive facilities. It is fundamental and all pervasive—it involves the whole of us right down to the cytoplasm of our cells. To return home is to find a world filled with beauty and a world to which we can belong. Everything seems to participate in a celestial harmony, grand in its purview yet utterly simple in its presence. We are greatly moved by the sheer beauty of it all while embracing and being embraced by a magnitude of order that cannot be specified. Because it is known without concepts, it is beyond words. Yet, it is utterly and conspicuously obvious to our feeling-nature. Homecoming is not just about cerebral free play. It is also about our upright body being released in gravity and dancing in the free play of verticality where our world makes sense and supports us as we make our way home. Homecoming is the event of embodiment, an event so close to us that we often need to be reminded of its importance.

First and foremost, holistic manual therapy is about coming home to our bodies, to the balanced integration of core and surface in the uplifted but grounded free play of our verticality in gravity. As Rolf repeatedly said, when the body is organized in gravity, gravity is no longer the enemy of the body but its liberator. We get in trouble when the order-thwarters are greater than the body's ability to freely and orthotropically appropriate gravity in the free play of the vertical. But when the organization of the body is improved upon, aches and pains begin to disappear, the conflicts and fixations that weigh us down begin to dissipate, and we begin to wake up to new possibilities for our life. Coming home is coming home to our bodies.

Kant's homecoming, while exposing our fundamental need for order, is just a bit too cerebral. In order to underscore the importance of the body, you could say that Rolf discovered the somatic secret of alchemy—a morphological imperative or somatic analog of the need for habitable orderliness and the means to bring it about. Comparing the art of Rolfing to how chemists determine the purity of substances, she says, "... if the angles are not sharp, show only sporadically, while the bulk of the material is ill-defined or amorphous, the chemist is warned that his substance needs further purification ..."[3] Analogously, as bodies approach integration in gravity through the shaping process of Rolfing, they take on a more and more integrated well-defined form, and, as a result, function more economically and exhibit easy, coordinated movement. The more well-defined the body becomes, the deeper one's experience of freedom, sense of place, and sense of belonging becomes.

When a body attains an integrated well-defined form, it manifests the beauty of normality: "And, when you see normal structure, all of a sudden you say, Why yes, of course, I recognize this as normal structure. Oddly enough, we all have intuitive appreciation of the normal. When we see something that is normal we say, Isn't that beautiful?, Doesn't he move beautifully? etc., etc. Nobody asks you to define that beauty, everybody recognizes it. It's an intuitive appreciation of normalcy."[4] Thus, we can say the homecoming consists of realizing the beauty of normalcy. To those who may be put off by the word "normal," remember that Rolf also said, "Average is not normal."

Conclusion

In our initial attempt to get a felt-sense of what holistic manual therapy is and what it aspires to, we saw that it was able to handle a great many of the physical complaints clients present. In addition, we uncovered a potential for self-discovery and growth. As a preliminary way to give voice to this potential, I likened it to a homecoming. Perhaps the most obvious but least appreciated feature of homecoming is that it is a bodily event.

Homecoming is coming home to my body at ease and free in a humanly habitable world. A body that feels at home, whose feeling-nature is free of conflict and fixation, and is at ease in an ever-changing world is a body integrated in gravity.

Élie Metchnikoff, the father of immunology, coined the word "ortho-biosis" to describe the ever-ongoing striving of life to improve upon and enhance itself and its circumstances. With respect to human beings ortho-biosis must also include orthotropism, the body's ever-present search for the vertical. As we begin to find integration in gravity our movement becomes more coordinated and less encumbered. We find ourselves danc-ing free in the integrated and grounded verticality of our upright bodies. Manual therapy is simply the conscious expression of these orthobiotic and orthotropic impulses toward our own enhancement. Orthobiosis also extends its reach to our environment. We can see the results of our ortho-biotic striving everywhere in our ceaseless shaping and improving upon of our environment. The word "radical" means "to return to the root." In that sense, manual therapy is the most radical approach to shaping and enhancing our selves. It goes to the source and works with the body's own strivings to enhance itself.

Living in a habitable world presupposes, of course, that there is a beautiful and habitable world that can be perceived. But sometimes the suffering is too much and we resort to armoring ourselves against the struggle with gravity and too many order-thwarters. We rigidify, den-sify, or make ourselves too soft in a futile attempt to protect ourselves. Unfortunately, such a defense makes it much more difficult to appreciate the beauty of the habitable world. When our body is in this kind of defended state, the beauty of the habitable literally makes no appreciable impression upon us—we become immune to being moved by beauty. Thus, it is no stretch of the imagination to say that manual therapy is the *conscious expression of orthobiosis.* Shaping the body and its relation to the environment through manual therapy is one of the most direct and powerful ways to make it possible to find our way home. The comfort of embodiment, the ability to feel at home and at ease almost anywhere, is an expression of the freedom that arises when we fully embrace where we already and always are.

In Chapter Eleven, we will return to the notions of embodiment and homecoming by investigating the experience of the seasoned manual therapist in love with his work. In an effort to further deepen our understanding of these matters, we will continue to uncover and elucidate their numinous dimension. In Chapter Eight we will introduce the idea that the body is sentient.

CHAPTER 2

The Territory

When I first began practicing Rolfing SI, I was excited and awed by the results I was getting. But soon the glow wore off and I began to question what I was doing. I was still getting good results, but I was worried about the formulistic way I was getting them. I had been trained, as all Rolfers had been trained, in how to apply Rolf's protocol of ten hour-long sessions, which she called "The Recipe." As a novice, I was certainly not prepared to work outside the dictates of the recipe. At the same time, I began to feel very mechanical in my approach, as if I were "Rolfing by numbers." At times I felt as though I was attempting to stamp all these individually different bodies into an external template. In order to learn how to work free of the recipe, I took a number of Rolfing SI workshops. But all I really learned were embellishments on the recipe.

Rolf created an astonishing system of holistic manual therapy and movement education designed to get the body right with itself and with gravity. Even though delivering therapy by following a formulistic protocol has some major drawbacks, the power of the recipe to help a great variety of clients is remarkable. If not one of a kind, the recipe is certainly a unique and clear example of something you rarely see—an extended step-by-step demonstration of how to reason and intervene holistically.

As you would expect, unlike her students, she could work often, easily, and without guilt outside her own recipe. Because she recognized the drawbacks of a formulistic approach, she embarked on creating an advanced training in the later years of her life. Unfortunately, she died before she could create a coherent non-formulistic approach to Rolfing SI. As a colleague once observed, she left the baby on the doorstep for us to raise.

Formulistic protocols by their very nature assume the existence of an ideal body or state that is assumed to constitute normality. The theory that there is an ideal structure that every body should strive to emulate can be called somatic idealism. Formulism and somatic idealism go hand in hand. Formulistic protocols dictate the same sequence of interventions in the same order. Even if they allow for some variation in how the interventions are sequenced, they necessarily presuppose the same outcome for every body. Since they assume the same outcome for every body, formulistic protocols surreptitiously perpetuate somatic idealism. Unfortunately, somatic idealism, whether it assumes an ideal form for the way the body should relate to gravity or an ideal notion of normality, does not work for everybody.

The other related drawback common to formulistic protocols is that they are sometimes incapable of attending to what is unique in each person. As a result, they are incapable of sequencing treatment strategies in the order required by each person's unique needs. Rolf understood the second drawback and did not always follow her own recipe. But she was less clear about somatic idealism and tended to use her idea of the ideal body as a standard against which to evaluate clients' bodies and the success of her work.

A good part of this book is devoted to how we raised the baby Rolf left on our doorstep. I soon discovered that the problems we faced were by no means unique to Rolfing SI. Our problems in raising our baby were the same problems that we face in every form of therapy. Even though the problems are not unique to Rolfing SI, they are much more acute primarily because practitioners are taught the work by means of a recipe they cannot do without. As a result, because our problems are more acute, they are easier to see. Nevertheless, all forms of therapy are at different stages of raising the same baby.

Around the time I was invited to train to be a teacher of Rolfing SI, I had been playing a little game with myself. During the course of working with clients, I would imagine that an omniscient therapist would appear demanding an explanation and justification for why I was working where

I was working. I was quite upset when I realized I could only give recipe answers, for example, "Don't work above the lumbodorsal junction during the sixth session."

The Omniscient Therapist

To highlight these issues, imagine we are following the omniscient therapist around as he is training practitioners during a workshop. The manual therapists are busily helping their clients when the omniscient therapist asks the entire class to think about how to explain and justify why they are working where they are working with their clients. He then asks for three students to volunteer. With some trepidation, a massage therapist raises her hand. She says that she is working on the hamstrings because they are tight. A biomechanical corrective therapist goes next and answers that he is working with a client's low back pain by freeing up a posteriorly torsioned sacrum. Lastly, a more eclectically trained therapist says that he is working according to the principle, *treat the worst first.*

After listening intently, the omniscient therapist looks at the massage therapist, and kindly says,

> "Well, yes, you are right, the hamstrings are tight. But there are at least twenty other tight places, why pick this one over them?" Then he turns to the biomechanically oriented therapist and asks, "Why address the posteriorly torsioned sacrum now when there is so much difficulty in his neck, rib cage, shoulder girdle, and cranium?" To the third therapist the omniscient therapist says, "You will see why later, but 'treat the worst first' is a strategy or tactic, not a principle. In this case, there are so many secondary fixations standing in the way that the primary one will not release until the secondary fixations do. Sometimes just the opposite is true. You may have to release the primary one before treating the secondary fixations. So how do you decide? Consider the possibility that there is more than just one serious restriction. What if there are five equally dysfunctional areas? Which one do you pick first?"

One last thing, how you work with your clients is very much based on how you conceive and practice your kind of therapy. What practice paradigm do you work in and what kind of results do you expect from your work? If your work is aimed at producing the relaxation response, it will not be capable of organizing the body of gravity or of releasing joint fixations. Swedish massage is an excellent way to bring about needed relaxation. But when it comes to releasing a bilaterally posteriorly fixed sacrum, relaxation-oriented therapy is not up to the job. If there are global patterns of strain in the body as a whole, employing techniques that relieve symptom by symptom without a grasp of the more global distortions will often produce poor results.

The Three Paradigms

The above reference to practice paradigms is my way of distinguishing among and categorizing the many forms of manual therapy. Called the *Three Paradigms of Practice*, it is meant to apply to any and all forms of healing and health care, whether the practitioners are surgeons, shamans, or hypnotists. Every form of health care you can imagine falls under one of three categories. The first paradigm is called the *relaxation* paradigm because its goal is to promote healing by relaxing the client. Examples include Swedish massage, hot/cold packs, hot tubs, etc. The second paradigm, the *corrective* paradigm rests upon a mechanomorphic theory (the view that the universe and all living things are mechanical events). Since corrective practitioners tend to think of the body as a soft machine made of parts, assessment and treatment are piecemeal and symptomatic. Practices that just adjust fixed joints, or limit themselves to one function or aspect of the body, such as lymph drainage, dentistry, or podiatry, qualify as corrective practices. The third approach is the *holistic* paradigm, which has as its goal integration, harmony, order, and the enhancement of function for the whole person. In addition, as Rolf well understood, the holistic paradigm is incomplete unless it includes getting the body right with its environment and gravity. We can sum up the goals of holism by means of a metaphor: holistic manual therapy tries to transform the sky, not push the stars. Some examples of the holistic approach are Eastern medicine, osteopathy, homeopathy, and Feldenkrais. The science and philosophy upon which holistic practices depend must also be holistic.

The three paradigms are hierarchically related to each other. The relaxation practitioner cannot attain the goals of the other two paradigms, except by accident. The corrective practitioner, as a matter of course, can achieve the goals of the relaxation paradigm but not the goals of the holistic paradigm, unless by accident. The holistic practitioner, as a matter of course, can achieve the goals of the first two paradigms. A pure practitioner of any one of the three paradigms is probably somewhat rare. With experience and practice many practitioners respond to the needs of their clients by working freely between all the paradigms. Also, it should be noted that manual therapy does not typically deal with disease.

These are differences that make a difference. For example, the second and third paradigm practitioners have very different views about biological order. Ignorance over the radically different way biological wholes and machines are ordered and respond to injury and intervention can muddy our assessments and limit our effectiveness. The important difference between how machines and living bodies are organized will be taken up in Chapter Eight.

The Three Questions

The order in which you treat a client is every bit as important as what you treat. As a result, a large part of this book will be devoted to understanding how therapy proceeds, why we do what we do, why we do it in the order we do, how we justify what we do, and what is the science and philosophy upon which they rest. As I struggled with the questions raised by confronting my imaginary omniscient therapist, it slowly dawned on me that at the core of everything we do sits three fundamental questions that must be asked and answered—not just by every manual therapist, but by every therapist. Furthermore, these questions must be asked at the beginning of every session, during every session, and at the end of the session or a series of sessions. They are: *what do I do first, what do I do next, and when am I finished?*

In an effort to answer these questions, I read book after book on the principles of manual therapy, went to conferences, met a lot of fine people, and talked to many famous authors, therapists, and teachers—and learned a lot. Feeling a bit like a second-rate Socrates, whenever I could reasonably do so I asked these three questions. There were many answers, but no really satisfactory ones. Strangely, from the answers I received, it seemed as if nobody had ever asked themselves these questions. There was much talk about principles, but little understanding of what was meant by principles or what meaning of principle was under consideration.

One unhelpful but humorous answer stands above the many I heard. I asked a well-known therapist and teacher why he just moved his hands from one place to another (why did he do what he did next?). He said, "I put my hands where my eyes drift to first." Apparently this worked for him, because he got great results with his clients. But it was a little too idiosyncratic to teach to other therapists. The question I didn't get a chance to ask him was how he knew that his eyes went to the right spot in the first place. Somehow he discovered a new assessment skill. If only he had taken the trouble to examine how he knew his eyes correctly went to the next place needing work, he could have developed a useful perceptual skill that could be taught to others.

As you might expect, most experienced practitioners tended to emphasize the importance of assessment when asked the three questions. Good assessment skills are crucial. Where you start, where you work next, and where and when you stop depends on your perceptual skills, your ability to perceive dysfunction, and when problems are released. If you cannot see what the problem is with your client, you cannot address it. The better you are able to perceive what your client needs, the better your work becomes. Rolf would often say to her students, "You are looking, but I want you to *see*."

Before we move on, I want to make two terminological points. Instead of talking about fixations, dysfunctional areas, or symptoms, I prefer the designation "order-thwarter" as a way of calling attention to the fact that order-thwarters are unified whole patterns that are involved with and compromise the organization and freedom of the whole person at many levels at once, from joints to worldviews. Therefore, I designate all fixations, whether they are found in our joints or worldviews as "order-thwarters."

Also, remember that the words "perception" and "seeing" when used in the context of this book are not limited to the visual. As we shall see, we are capable of seeing with our feeling-nature and energy, for example. Manipulating soft tissue is a form of perception. And when all is said and done, we will come to understand that the entire body is the sensorium.

We will look at the nature of perception in Chapter Six and how to train it in Chapter Seven.

Types of Assessment and Intervention

Accurate and comprehensive client assessment is essential to effective intervention, especially when working with the whole person. Since knowing what to look for in the way of order-thwarters precedes treatment, in order to assist the development of the practitioner's perceptual skills, I identified and developed five interrelated types of assessment and intervention (I originally called them the five taxonomies of assessment). In addition to their practical application, the great number of actual and potential ways to assess and treat that are represented in these five types also reveals quite clearly the breadth and depth of holistic manual therapy.

The five types are as follows: 1) *Structural Assessment and Intervention* is concerned with assessing structure and organizing it by employing a variety of structural techniques that include myofascial techniques (some of which are unique to Rolfing SI) as well as techniques that affect the organs, craniosacral system, and nerves; 2) *Geometric Assessment and Intervention* is similar to the structural type but locates structural strains and imbalances and their resolution in terms of geometric patterns and forms; 3) *Functional Assessment and Intervention* targets recognizing and resolving dysfunctional patterns of movement, and promoting normal coordinated movement by means of a variety of manipulation and movement techniques; 4) *Energy Assessment and Intervention* is concerned with recognizing dysfunctional energy patterns and how to use energy techniques to directly facilitate structural integrity as well as cultivate a perceptual acuity to the resident fields within and surrounding the body; and 5) *Psychobiological Orientation (or Intentionality) Assessment and Intervention* is concerned with the recognition and resolution of emotional fixations, worldview conflicts, trauma, and other similar difficulties that undermine structure and an individual's orientation to the world.

Since the structural, geometric, functional assessments, and interventions are probably more familiar, we won't spend a lot of time on them. But the energy and psychobiological orientation types, each for different reasons, need a little more elucidation.

Since the idea of the psychobiological orientation (or intentionality) assessment and intervention category is not well known, but important to holistic manual therapy, we will devote Chapter Five to laying out what it is and offering a number of case histories to illustrate what it is and how it works. The rest of this chapter will be devoted to a short elucidation of the energy assessment/intervention category and an introduction to the principles of intervention. Chapters Three and Four will complete the discussion of principles.

Energy Work

Manual therapy and energy work have always had a surreptitious relationship. Even though they work together, they often don't trust each other. Most biologists believe that the idea of vital energy is a fiction on the order of phlogiston. Rolf was interested in energy and its role in her work from the very beginning. But she did not teach or emphasize it. In the intervening years following her death, interest in energy work has exploded. Today, there are a large number of classes and workshops being offered in energy work around the world. Since it is part of the territory of manual therapy and has been so for thousands of years, it deserves a showing.

Modern physics defines energy as "the capacity for work." For the sake of clarity and in contrast to the way physics defines energy, we will refer to the energy familiar to the energy practitioner as *phenomenological energy*. It is fair to say that the capacity for work captures a feature common to all forms of energy, including what we are calling phenomenological energy. Beyond that, however, it falls impossibly short as both a definition and a description of phenomenological energy and how it functions in healing. It misses entirely the central role of experience in our understanding and use of vital energy. Unlike the capacity for work, phenomenological energy can be felt directly by both the practitioner and client. This ability to experience and perceive phenomenological energy depends on the ability of the practitioner to expand his or her perceptual abilities to include a whole-body understanding. The ability to perceive phenomenological energy in all its variegated activities is critical to the practitioner's ability to deliver effective therapy. Without it, proper assessment and treatment are limited.

Phenomenological energy is a perceivable, self-organizing, sentient intelligence responsible for sustaining and maintaining life. For it to manifest in a healing session, a change in the orientation (intentionality) of the practitioner is absolutely essential. In a very real sense, the first intervention of any healing session consists of the practitioner getting rid of his or her own conflicts and fixations as well as any willful desire to help or heal. By getting out of the way, the practitioner enters a potent state of allowing that enables him or her to clear a space within which phenomenological energy can do its work. When phenomenological energy appears, the practitioner is infused with the capacity or power to promote healthy change.

Written by one who knows where of he speaks, here is an example of an ancient Taoist text encouraging us to cultivate inner power:

1. When your body is not aligned,
2. The inner power will not come.
3. When you are not tranquil within,

4. Your mind will not be well ordered.
5. Align your body, assist the inner power,
6. it will gradually come on its own.[5]

Even if practitioners, now and then, employ non-energy techniques during energy sessions, they are likely to be infused automatically with the same energy and become more effective. Even though the great majority of energy practitioners use touch-based techniques to affect change, proximity to the body is not essential. The effects of energy healing and the relationship between the practitioner and client are at bottom nonlocal.*

Some of the many ways phenomenological energy appears to both client and practitioner are as follows: as pressure or fullness in the area being worked on, tingling, flowing both inside and around the body, a sense that something is constantly working at freeing up some restriction or other, fittingness of the body's personal geometry with the surrounding energy environment and its geometry, fluid and/or somewhat stationary geometric shapes that are difficult to describe struggling to right themselves inside and outside the body, an exacerbation of symptoms followed by a release, reorganization at all levels of the person, various biodynamic tidal phenomena, and many more.

Principles

Now that we have explored the territory of holistic manual therapy, it is necessary to get a preliminary understanding of the principles of intervention. An experienced therapist knows how to recognize many types of dysfunction and how to release them. But how does this therapist take all the information gathered from assessments and formulate a treatment strategy? Every choice you make as to where you will begin, where you will work next, and when you will finish must have some basis or reason for your choosing it. The beginning Rolfer's answer is simple but hardly

---

*For more on this topic, see my book *Mind Body Zen* (Berkeley: North Atlantic Books, 2010).

helpful—follow the recipe. It is also not useful or helpful to know that you work by intuition. Intuition is notoriously difficult to define and teach. Accordingly, this book represents the attempt to create a viable decision-making process based on the principles of intervention. I am not suggesting you give up your intuition. Instead of being suspicious of intuition, we should learn to cultivate and clarify it. It turns out that the three-step exercise I developed in Chapters Six and Seven for training perception will also train and sharpen your intuition.

To get an idea of what principles are and how they function, consider a rather different context. John Cage, a wild and wonderfully creative contemporary American composer who invented and explored aleatory music with a kind of Zen-like excess, relates an interesting story that elegantly illustrates the relevant use of the word "principle." Cage knew and studied with many of the great artists of the twentieth century. The following story comes from when he studied with Arnold Schoenberg, creator of the twelve-tone system of composition.

> During a counterpoint class at UCLA, Schoenberg sent everybody to the blackboard. We were to solve a particular problem he had given and to turn around when finished so that he could check on the correctness of the solution. I did as directed. He said, "That's good. Now find another solution." I did. He said, "Another." Again I found one. Again he said, "Another." And so on. Finally, I said, "There are no more solutions." He said, "What is the principle underlying all of the solutions?"[6]

Many different uses and definitions of the word "principle" can be found in philosophical treatises and scientific investigations. The word "principle" can refer to a basic law, a fundamental property, or a value. But the one relevant to our discussion defines a principle as a fundamental rule from which something proceeds, such as a chain of reasoning. For example, even though a simple series like "2, 4, 6, 8 . . ." can be continued without much thought, its continuation is based on a principle: "to continue the series add two to the last number." Analogously, in the case of manual therapy, the principles of intervention are fundamental rules from which a clinical decision-making process proceeds. When Schoenberg asks "What is the principle underlying all of the solutions?" he clearly demonstrates this use.

If we expand the lesson learned in Cage's story to the clinical decision-making process, we can see that the solutions Cage produced for Schoenberg are analogous to the many treatment strategies one might use to resolve back pain in a number of different clients. The strategies by which one approaches each patient's back pain can be as varied as the patients themselves. Like Cage we may not at first fully realize how our formulation of treatment strategies is guided by principles, but realize it or not, principles are what allow us to find solutions and create strategies. In the clinical setting strategies function like rules of thumb—they cannot apply in all cases. By their very nature, rules of thumb are rules that can be broken. In the hands of an experienced practitioner, they are formulated and abandoned to suit the individual needs of each patient. However, because principles underlie all strategies and solutions, because they are what allow us to form any given strategy or solution in the first place, they cannot be abandoned, even creatively. In fact, once we understand that principles are like the rules that define a game, it makes no sense to abandon them.

Recall the three questions we must always ask when formulating a treatment strategy. No matter how we arrive at our answers—whether from intuition, from following a formulistic protocol, from just treating symptom by symptom, or from applying principles—these questions are presupposed in every single clinical decision we make whether we bring them to consciousness or not. The extent to which these questions are not asked, are avoided, or not properly answered is why patients often suffer from inappropriate therapy. Explicitly or tacitly, every therapeutic decision we make and every attempt to sequence our decisions into appropriate treatment strategies display, for good or ill, how well we have answered these three questions. If our interventions are to avoid becoming nothing more than mere symptom chasing or blind adherence to formulistic protocols, we must understand the nature of the principles of intervention and how they function in the clinical decision-making process.

Other factors that contribute to our clinical decision-making process besides principles and good assessment skills include research data about how patients respond to various treatment protocols; functional outcome measurements; a more than adequate understanding of anatomy, physiology, and kinesiology; contraindications; and development of good technical skills. A moment's reflection shows, however, that even if we have mastered all of these factors and more, we still need some rational way to prioritize all of this information, decide what is relevant given the unique needs and limitations of each patient, and then sequence our decisions into an appropriate program of treatment. This ability to prioritize information into a treatment strategy comes from a tacit or explicit understanding of principles.

CHAPTER 3

In Search of Principles

A great deal of cross-disciplinary agreement exists about the importance of principles. Even a cursory glance at the many articles and books written in the disciplines of pain management, osteopathy, physical therapy, chiropractic, Rolfing SI, and many other related disciplines reveals repeated references to principles coupled with the recognition of the need for a rational decision-making process. The word "principle" is very popular in the literature and often shows up in article and book titles. Indeed, one of the root meanings of the word "rational" is "to think in accordance with principles." Oddly enough, however, none of the numerous discussions ever address the most basic of questions: what is a principle and what constitutes a principle of intervention? As a direct result of not clarifying what kinds of principles are at issue, very few of these texts ever come close to stating a single principle of intervention. In fact, often what passes for principles in the literature are not principles at all. When principles are actually stated, they turn out not to be the principles of intervention, but the principles of some other related endeavor. Therefore, a coherent and clinically meaningful discussion of principles is difficult to find. This chapter is aimed at clarifying these confusions around principles and spelling out in some detail their role in clinical decision making.

Principles and Strategies

Conflating principles with strategies is by far the most common error. Many authors mistakenly think they are articulating the principles of intervention when, in fact, they are simply laying out a number of effective treatment strategies or protocols designed to treat local somatic dysfunctions. Osteopath Philip Greenman's excellent book, *Principles of Manual Medicine*, consistently exemplifies this confusion. He says for example, "In treating dysfunctions of the rib cage there are principles of treatment which should be followed for the best result. Almost without exception, one should make a structural diagnosis and manual medicine treatment to the thoracic spine prior to addressing the ribs individually or in groups."[7] While this recommendation for treatment makes good clinical sense and is true most of the time, it is not a principle of intervention or treatment. It is, rather, a treatment strategy or tactic. If it were a principle, one would not be able to say "almost without exception." Strategies can be abandoned according to the individual needs and responses of the patient. But since principles are the basis on which we formulate further treatment strategies, since they behave like the rules that define the game of manual therapy, they cannot be abandoned. If you abandon a principle of intervention, it is analogous to abandoning the rules that define a game. If you abandon a rule or rules that define a game, you are no longer playing the game. Clearly, a chain of reasoning cannot be based on strategy rules. As a result, Greenman's belief that he has stated a principle is mistaken.

Doctors R. C. Schafer and L. J. Faye, in a book that purports to be about the principles of dynamic chiropractic, also exemplify a similar confusion. In the introductory chapter, they broach the question of principles and claim, "This section will attempt to briefly define certain general principles that underlie most all chiropractic adjustive techniques, yet few apply in all instances. These principles must be amended to the situation at hand and the individual making the application."[8] Like so many authors who conflate treatment strategies with principles, they mistakenly conclude that principles must be amended to the situation at hand. Not surprisingly, their discussion of principles is not about principles at all. It is actually about other related issues like the goal of therapy, technique, table height, proper positioning of the hands in applying techniques, and other practical considerations not relevant to delineating the principles of intervention.

Principles and Normal Function

Another common confusion occurs when theorists point to well established observations about normal body functioning and call them principles. These so-called principles are more analogous to what we might call the laws of normal function. The Principle of the Artery, as many osteopaths refer to it, is a good example of this mistake. It is not a principle of intervention but a law of normal functioning. Being able to recognize and return the body to normal function is, of course, an important prerequisite for becoming a competent therapist. Normal function is, after all, one of the most important goals of all therapy. But the goal of normal or enhanced function is not a principle of intervention. Schafer and Faye make the same mistake when they include a discussion of the goal of therapy in a section devoted to principles. Clearly, however, the goals of therapy are quite different in kind from the principles of intervention. Therapeutic goals are achieved by means of the appropriate application of principles and sequencing of interventions—goals are not self-generating principles on the basis of which strategies are formulated.

Two Senses of Principle

Another common mistake involves confusing the principles of other related endeavors with the principles of intervention. This mistake can often be found in the psychological literature where theorists are concerned with stating the principles governing the therapeutic relationship. Ron Kurtz, PhD, calls one of these principles the *Principle of Nonviolence*. It requires that the clinician not use force when working with clients in order to achieve a therapeutic result. He says, "Violence in therapy is very subtle...When someone simply assumes they know what is best for others, you have violence...When therapists ask questions to gather information for themselves, often interrupting the client to do so, that's violence, and it breeds resistance...Nonviolence is born of an attitude of acceptance and an active attention to the way events naturally unfold."[9] While such discussions are extremely important and relevant to the practice of all health care professionals, these sorts of principles are not the same as the principles of intervention. Gaining awareness of one's own psychological states, being open and accepting of our clients, and generally knowing how to create the proper client/practitioner relationship is supremely important for the success of all therapy. Clearly, however, knowing how to create the proper environment for therapy will not provide the necessary guidelines for deciding how to intervene in any given case.

Principles, Evaluation, and Technique

Often theorists believe they are articulating the principles of intervention when in fact they are discussing the importance of evaluation, outcome assessment, or the proper application of techniques. Under a section entitled "Principles of Myofascial Release Treatment" Robert Ward lists thirteen principles. Not one of the principles listed, however, is a principle of intervention. Principle 4, for example, says, "Palpatory evaluations should test the same sites passively, because passive testing gives more accurate information."[10] This statement is not a principle of intervention but a recommendation on how to conduct a proper evaluation on the basis of an important observation about palpation. Fred Mitchell Jr. notes that the concepts of Muscle Energy manual therapy "are so interrelated that a linear exposition of principles is difficult." Nevertheless, he goes on to say that his "basic principles are the same for all passive joints: voluntary muscle contractions are exerted against a precisely executed counter force to loosen the specifically localized joints for passive articulation during postcontraction relaxation."[11] As important as this observation is, what Mitchell has stated is not a principle of intervention but a recommendation for and description of how to apply a particular technique.

Principles and Philosophy

Another common mistake involves confusing the principles of intervention with a statement of the philosophy of a particular discipline. Actually, these so-called statements of philosophy are not even examples of true philosophy, but merely pronouncements of the values that particular disciplines believe their practitioners should embrace. Examples of these values are: "Do no harm," "Empower the patient to be responsible for his or her own well-being," and so on. Few would deny that espousing and adhering to such values is important. But once again, adhering to these values will not provide us with a way to sequence our clinical decisions and create appropriate treatment strategies.

Game Analogy

Geoffrey D. Maitland comes the closest to understanding the nature of principles when he compares manipulation to certain kinds of games. He says, "Manipulation is not like a game of golf where the player uses a technique to hit a ball in the direction he wants it to go, although most people tend to use the techniques of manipulation this way... Manipulation is more like a game of chess... An even better analogy is a game of Contract Bridge... the technique of playing the cards requires considered, careful planning."[12] He also says, "The reasoning and planning in the application of techniques are the *sin qua non*, not the techniques *per se*."[13]

Even though G. D. Maitland correctly understands the relevance of the game analogy to the process of formulating the "right sequence of priority," he does not grasp what a principle of intervention is. In fact he never discusses the principles of intervention at all. Because he never sees the point of discussing the principles of intervention, he cannot fully grasp the "reasoning and planning in the application of techniques" that he correctly recognizes as so important. Instead of laying out the principles that form the basis of the reasoning and planning involved in formulating strategies and tactics, he devotes himself to elaborating a precise examination process. His assessments belong under the structural and functional categories.

There can be no question about the importance of G. D. Maitland's contribution to our understanding of how to perform a proper assessment. The extent to which a clinician is unable to gather the relevant information about the patient's condition is the extent to which the clinician must be incapable of formulating an adequate treatment strategy. After gathering all the relevant information from the examination process, however, if the clinician has neither an explicit nor tacit understanding of the principles of intervention, the clinician has no rational basis for how he or she sequences the application of techniques. Principles, as we shall see, are like the rules that define the nature of a game. A player or clinician cannot engage in the careful, considered planning that G. D. Maitland correctly deems so important, if he or she does not know or understand the rules of the game or the principles of intervention. And it is these rules that G. D. Maitland never articulates.

In pointing out the above mistakes, I do not want to be misunderstood as suggesting that these factors are not important or are somehow irrelevant to how we make clinical decisions and formulate strategies. Obviously, being able to evaluate somatic dysfunction, recognize normal function, state the goals of therapy, appropriately apply a wide range of techniques, assess functional outcomes, and create the proper client/practitioner relationship all occupy an important place in the clinical decision-making process. The important point is, however, that without an explicit or tacit understanding of the principles of intervention, these factors taken by themselves or collectively give us no clear and rational way to decide what to do first, what to do next, and when to finish.

Two Kinds of Rules

Given all the confusions in the literature over principles and that no one has wrestled with the question of what constitutes a principle, it is not surprising that we find a great deal of ambiguity in every attempt to sequence clinical decisions into appropriate treatment strategies. Because these issues about principles are so critically important to what clinicians do, day in and day out, it behooves us to understand what a principle is before we try to state the principles of intervention.

As I stated, the relevant meaning of the concept of "principle" is a rule on the basis of which a chain of reasoning or clinical decision-making process proceeds. An easy way to grasp what a principle is and how it functions is to consider a simple game. In a game of checkers, we can distinguish between two kinds of rules: constitutive rules and strategy rules. Constitutive rules are the rules that define how the game is played. Since the constitutive rules define the game itself, breaking one or more of these rules is tantamount to no longer playing the game. If one of the players moves his or her piece off the board and onto the table to avoid losing, the player is not exhibiting great gamesmanship and creativity but quite simply no longer playing checkers.

Strategy rules, in contrast, are rules of thumb. They do not define the game. Rather, they state generalities based on experience about which moves are most often considered the best under certain recurring situations. Unlike constitutive rules, breaking a strategy rule does not imply that one is no longer playing the game. "Always" and "never" cannot under any circumstances apply to strategy rules. If a beginning player loses because he or she consistently breaks strategy rules, we would see the player as an inexperienced opponent. We would not accuse him or her of no longer playing checkers. If we were to observe a player who always wins at checkers, but breaks many strategy rules, we would not conclude that the player is no longer playing checkers or that he or she is a poor player. We would conclude that the player is a highly skilled, creative, and experienced player.

In the holistic paradigm, the principles of therapeutic intervention function much like the constitutive rules of a game; strategies and tactics function like rules of thumb. Unlike strategies, principles define the therapeutic arena and state the conditions under which normal and enhanced function occur. Unlike strategies and tactics, they are small in number and under consideration every time we attempt to intervene or formulate a treatment plan. Like the constitutive rules of a game, they cannot be cast aside at the discretion of the practitioner. However, the principles of intervention are unlike constitutive rules of a game in two important ways: they state the necessary, but not sufficient, conditions under which normal or enhanced function is obtained, and they are not stated in temporal language like strategies, tactics, and rules of thumb are. Strategies and tactics say, "Do X before Y"; principles say "X is a function or condition of Y" and leave it entirely open as to whether X or Y should be done first. Just as breaking any rule that defines a game amounts to no longer playing the game, ignoring or casting aside any principle of intervention amounts to no longer engaging in the holistic approach to somatic therapy.

Strategies and tactics state the temporal order in which interventions are to be applied, and principles state the basis upon which this temporal order is formulated. Therefore, any time we discover a statement that purports to be a principle but contains temporal language, we can assume that it is probably a strategy rule masquerading as a principle. Greenman's recommendation that one should resolve thoracic facet restrictions *before* dealing with rib dysfunctions is a good example of the temporal order that all strategies and tactics display. Clearly, Greenman is articulating a strategy rule, not a principle of intervention, as he thinks. Greenman's rule is an example of a strategy rule that applies most of the time. However, no matter how applicable such strategy rules generally are and no matter how many of them a practitioner knows, further strategies and tactics cannot be based on them. Strategies and tactics always permit exceptions. They can neither be the basis for making exceptions or for formulating further strategies. Only principles function that way.

Recall our discussion of the corrective paradigm and notice that the corrective practitioner only has strategy rules at his or her disposal. The principles of intervention are the principles of a holistic system and cannot be used in the second paradigm. Thus, the corrective practitioner has no way to formulate a treatment plan. As a result, therapeutic intervention becomes an intuitive hit-or-miss affair always poised on the brink of falling into formulism or symptom chasing. And neither of these two methods is properly attentive to the way clients change in response to treatment. Let's look at this point more carefully.

To many practitioners the claim that principles cannot be amended to the particular needs of the patient must sound strange, if not excessive. The problem, however, is not with this claim, but with confusion over what principles are and how they function in holistic thinking. If the nature of principles is not properly understood, there will be a tendency to confuse principles with statements that are not principles, as we have already seen. Principles are regularly confused with strategies, the goals of therapy, the "laws" of normal function, the principles of some other related endeavor like the therapeutic relationship, the philosophical values of a particular discipline, and so forth. Because many of these non-principles can be amended or cast aside during therapy and because many of them are somewhat debatable, it is not at all surprising that practitioners conclude that principles can sometimes be abandoned.

With these confusions hovering in the background, Grodin and Cantu in an article on soft tissue mobilization lay out what they think are the "Principles of Treatment Application." Unfortunately, their purported principles are, for the most part, a list of strategies and techniques and a recommendation for a sequence of interventions for which no principled justification is given. Why should we follow this five-step plan in this order as opposed to any other? What is the basis (principle) for these choices? They say, "Once the pathology has been identified by examination, appropriate goals are set and a soft tissue approach used as necessary... The proper sequence of the patient should ideally consist of:

1. Soft tissue mobilization to the area of hypomotility,
2. Joint mobilization following normalization of the soft tissue,
3. Soft tissue elongation based on the new range of motion,
4. Neuromuscular reeducation to restore normal movement to the area of aberrant motion,

5. Home program to maintain the increase in range of motion, quality of movement, and to remove lever arms and fulcruming on the area of aberrant motion."[14]

Confusing rules that lay out a temporal treatment sequence with principles is quite common in the corrective paradigm. Rules such as "treat the worst first" and other similar rules of thumb are clearly strategy rules that focus only on treating the local and related areas of dysfunction while ignoring the overall response of the whole body. This way of working and thinking is typical of the corrective approach. Since rules of thumb are not principles, they cannot be the logical basis for generating further strategy rules. Since they cannot be the basis for formulating strategies, no coherent or rational decision-making process can proceed from them.

By way of illustration, let us imagine that the examination process and the above rules lead a practitioner to treat a patient's low back. Strategies and tactics designed to release local areas associated with the client's back pain will produce good results if the whole body can support and adapt to the manipulations. If the whole body cannot adapt or support the local manipulations, then either the local area will revert to its dysfunctional state or strain will be driven elsewhere, sometimes exacerbating other dysfunctional areas. Predictably, if the patient does not get better or new problems show up elsewhere in the body, or other dysfunctional areas worsen, the practitioner who follows such rules is often at a loss to understand what is happening and how to proceed next. At such turning points, if we have no principles to guide us, we are easily led into either blindly casting about for other strategies or continuing the same ineffective treatment protocol session after session. Obviously neither method is likely to produce the desired results.

Since the corrective approach by its very nature is fundamentally incapable of recognizing how injury and local interventions affect the whole body, it is logically impossible to formulate a coherent set of principles to guide treatment within the corrective paradigm. If a corrective practitioner were to embrace a non-mechanistic understanding of living form, the practitioner would be led to see the body as a unified whole that responds as a whole to injury or intervention. If the practitioner were also to understand the importance of gravity to how the body compensates around an injury and supports or fails to support any intervention, he or she would be led to a richer and fuller understanding of how the exquisite deliquescence of the whole soma responds to imbalance, injury, or intervention.

We are seeing that more and more manual therapists are beginning to wake up to the importance of Rolf's insights into gravity. "Even experienced clinicians will enhance their clinical acumen by widening their perspective to recognize gravity as a systemic stressor and expanding their diagnostic examination to look for dysfunction in parts of the pattern not previously considered."[15] Bolstered by this richer understanding, logic and experience would necessarily lead the practitioner in the direction of the holistic paradigm. He or she would soon realize no principle of intervention can be fulfilled unless all are. As a consequence, the practitioner would be forced to conclude that a purely corrective approach cannot provide a rational basis for clinical decision making because it cannot be based, implicitly or explicitly, on a coherent or complete set of principles.

Given all the confusions surrounding the nature of principles and the holistic paradigm, we should not be surprised by the prevalent but mistaken belief that principles can be amended according to the individual needs of the patient. Nevertheless, these observations about the corrective paradigm should not lead us to conclude that corrective practices have no place in the clinical setting. Many times a corrective approach is enough to resolve a patient's dysfunction. Any further attempt to pursue a holistic approach in such a case may be a waste of time, especially if the patient is only interested in restoring function and has no interest in enhancing function. However, the ability to decide whether a holistic or corrective approach is appropriate for any given client, in principle, cannot be properly decided from within the framework of the corrective paradigm. The decision must come from a practitioner who understands how living wholes function and adapt, and who can practice in both the corrective and holistic paradigms. Nevertheless, clinical experience shows that more times than not restoration of function is not possible without the more thorough non-formulistic holistic approach.*

Necessary and Sufficient Conditions

In order to fully understand how the principles of intervention function in the clinical setting, we must first understand how necessary and sufficient conditions function. A necessary condition is a condition or set of conditions without which a phenomenon could not occur. A sufficient condition is a condition or set of conditions that, if present, are enough to guarantee that a phenomenon will occur. Oxygen, for example, is a necessary condition of fire. Without the presence of oxygen, fire is not possible. If oxygen were a sufficient condition, its mere presence would be enough to create fire. Since the mere presence of oxygen all by itself is not enough to create a fire, it is a necessary but not sufficient condition.

For the purposes of illustrating how necessary conditions function let us look at what we call the Principle of Adaptability. The adaptability principle is based on the observation and understanding that the body is a highly adaptable and plastic living whole. When the body is injured, say in an automobile accident, it often develops patterns of compensation in relation to the original pattern of injury. The automobile accident does not just cause a local problem with some "part" of the body, it creates global patterns of strain that in turn affects the organization and functioning of the whole body in gravity. The original pattern of injury more often than not is laid down on other previous injuries and postural imbalances. Along with the resulting patterns of compensation in relation to gravity, these imbalances and injury patterns result in a complicated loss of plasticity

---

*For two studies that illustrate these points in detail, see John Cottingham and Jeffrey Maitland's following articles: "A Three-Paradigm Treatment Model Using Soft Tissue Mobilization and Guided Movement—Awareness Techniques for a Patient with Chronic Low Back Pain: A Case Study," *Journal of Orthopedic and Sports Physical Therapy* 26, no. 3 (1997): 155–167; "Integrating Manual and Movement Therapy with Philosophical Counseling for Treatment of a Patient with Amyotrophic Lateral Sclerosis: A Case Study That Explores the Principles of Holistic Intervention," *Alternative Therapies in Health and Medicine* 6, no. 2 (2000): 120–127.

and adaptability throughout the entire body. Over time further losses in movement, plasticity, and adaptability will appear as the body struggles with gravity in its daily activities. If these complicated patterns of strain and compensation are not released in the proper order, the body will not be able to respond properly to interventions designed to release the original injury site or any other area of dysfunction.

Adaptability is clearly important in any conceivable clinical setting— every attempt to restore or enhance function must take account of whether the body can adapt to any proposed strategy of intervention. If the body cannot adapt to an intervention or series of interventions, then either it will revert to its dysfunctional state or further strain will be driven to other areas of the body, or both. If the body is completely incapable of adapting to any possible strategy within a particular form of therapy, then the system of therapy is incapable of treating the patient's somatic dysfunction and some other therapy must be found. Thus, the Principle of Adaptability says "any attempt to restore or enhance normal function is a function of the body's ability to adapt to the intervention." The principle does not say that preparing the body to adapt to an intervention must always precede every attempt to restore or enhance function, only that adaptability is a necessary condition of appropriate intervention.

In much the same way that oxygen is a necessary condition of fire, the ability of the body to adapt to any intervention is a necessary condition of restoring or enhancing function. We can state a principle of the art of starting fires as "Starting a fire is a function of the presence of oxygen." If we are trying to start a fire and oxygen is present, then the principle is fulfilled and we can start our fire. Similarly, if we decide that we must manipulate a pelvic upslip, a posteriorly torsioned sacrum, and a type II dysfunction of L4 on L5 in order to relieve a patient's back pain, and the body can adapt to our proposed manipulative strategy, then the principle is fulfilled. All things being equal, we can then proceed to the application of our techniques. If the body cannot adapt to our proposed strategy, then we must prepare the body in precisely those areas where it cannot adapt. If the patient is too ill to respond or for other reasons incapable of significantly adapting to the proposed type of somatic therapy, then some other form of therapy must be found.

Depending upon the degree of adaptability in our client's body, preparatory work can occur either before, after, or at the same time we manipulate the areas associated with the client's back pain. If adaptability were a sufficient condition, then we would be required to prepare the body to receive our manipulations each and every time we intervened. But obviously such a requirement is too strong. Thus, the principles of intervention state the necessary conditions under which normal and enhanced function can appear. Since the principles do not state sufficient conditions, it is clear that other conditions must also be fulfilled for normal or enhanced function to appear, such as a skilled and knowledgeable therapist, a willing patient who shows up for appointments, a good evaluation of the patient, and so on. With these considerations in mind, let us turn to the principles.

CHAPTER 4

The Principles of Intervention

The principles of intervention must reflect the nature of biological order, not the way machines are ordered. Living bodies are not soft machines created from pre-shaped parts. Rather, they are developmental wholes. They are self-shaping, self-organizing, self-sensing, seamless unified wholes in which no one aspect or relation is more important to the organization of the whole than the whole itself. As a way to begin thinking about the relationship between principles and biological order, consider an analogy from Merleau-Ponty: "In a soap bubble as in an organism, what happens at each point is determined by what happens at all others. But this is the definition of order."[16] This kind of order characterizes living wholes and is at the heart and the foundation of any holistic form of therapy. It demands of the practitioner the ability to think and perceive holistically. Just as every part of the body is a reflection of the whole, every principle reflects the others. They are variations of each other, and no one principle is applicable in isolation from the others. The holistic principle is the overarching principle that governs all the others; it states how they function together in relation to each other.

HOLISTIC PRINCIPLE

No principle can be fulfilled completely unless all principles
are fulfilled completely.

Because the holistic principle governs and states how the principles of intervention function together in a holistic system, it is properly called a *meta-principle.* Since principles are the basis for clinical decision making, any intervention, session, or series of sessions always involves the reciprocal application and understanding of all the principles at once. The fundamental principle of holistic intervention is reflected in Merleau-Ponty's soap bubble analogy, "what happens at each point is determined by what happens at all others."

Every intervention or series of interventions requires a thorough examination and evaluation of the client across the five categories (or taxonomies) of assessment that includes a determination of which principles are fulfilled and how well or poorly they are fulfilled in each category of assessment. All strategies and tactics are formulated on the basis of how well or poorly each principle is fulfilled within the whole person. All principles must be applied in terms of what is morphologically appropriate and possible for each individual client in relation to his or her unique set of changing and unchanging limitations and in relation to gravity and the environment.

ADAPTABILITY PRINCIPLE

Integration is a function of the whole person's ability to appropriately adapt to ever changing internal and external environments.

Any attempt to bring the whole person to a new level of integration is a function of the whole person's ability to appropriately adapt to any intervention or series of interventions. If the whole person is unable to adapt to any intervention or series of interventions, then 1) the soma will revert to its pre-intervention state of disorder, dysfunction, or disease, 2) strain and disorder will be driven elsewhere in the system, or 3) both events will occur.

SUPPORT PRINCIPLE

Integration is a function of available support.

The Support Principle is a specific application of the Adaptability Principle. It rests on the recognition that spacetime, environment, and gravity are equiprimordial relationships within which the whole person participates and to which the whole person is related. The organization and integration of our psychobiological orthotropic nature is a function of not only how the whole is related to itself but also how the whole is related to and appropriates gravity and the environment. The extent to which higher levels of order are possible is the extent to which the whole person finds support within the limitations of spacetime, gravity, and the environment.

One of Rolf's most important contributions to somatic therapy was the recognition that the ever present force of gravity has a profound effect on how the body accommodates to all somatic imbalance and all injury. She also realized that support in gravity is critical to any attempt to correct or enhance the structure and functioning of the body. If a practitioner attempts to correct facet restrictions in the spine, for example, and the legs do not properly support the upper body, then the intervention will drive the strain elsewhere, sometimes worsening other dysfunctional areas, and/or the spine will revert to its dysfunctional state.

The Support Principle is Rolf's gravity principle. It is more specific than the adaptability principle because it emphasizes how the body adapts or fails to adapt to the ever present influence of gravity.

CONTINUITY PRINCIPLE

Integration is a function of appropriate continuity

Like the Support Principle, *the Continuity Principle is a specific application of the Adaptability Principle.* Loss of appropriate continuity compromises healthy functioning and normal coordinated activity. Functional integrity, configural identity, systemic coherence, and hierarchical organization manifest in appropriate continuity throughout every level of the whole person as described by the five categories of assessment. All somas, since they are alive, exhibit some degree of continuity. A soma's degree of continuity and coherence is a function of its freedom from dysfunction and hence a function of its freedom to orthotropically appropriate gravity by organizing around its midline.

PALINTONIC PRINCIPLE

Integration is a function of palintonic harmony.

Palintonicity appears with the manifestation of orthogonal relationships (e.g., horizontal and vertical lines/planes intersecting at right angles in the X, Y, and Z axis or the sagittal, coronal, and transverse planes). The appearance of horizontals at the joints and normal coordinated movement arise together. As a person approaches somatic integration, palintonic harmony begins to appear throughout the whole person in relation to the environment as described by the five categories of assessment.

The success of any intervention or series of interventions is a function of appropriate spatial relationships—for example, back/front, side/side, top/bottom, inside/outside, and orthogonal balance. Palintonic harmony describes the spatial, somatic geometry of order, which is so apparent as a body approaches somatic integration. It expresses the unity of opposition that arises among all structures, spaces, volumes, and planes of an integrated soma as it moves through space. It describes the unity of opposition or balanced tension that exists when back/front, inside/outside, side/side, and up/down relationships approach balance with respect to each other and gravity. Palintonic harmony also describes the unity of opposition that arises among all aspects of the whole person as described by the five categories as the whole person approaches integration. *The extent to which any of these relationships is established is a function of how well all of them are established in relation to gravity and the environment.*

Palintonos is a Greek word. It was used by the great pre-Socratic philosopher Heraclitus (*c.* 500 BCE) in the following aphorism: "They do not apprehend how in differing with itself it is brought to agree with itself:

palintonic harmony, like that of the bow and the lyre." *Palintonos* literally means "stretched back and forth." It means, therefore, the unity of opposition or balanced tension.

CLOSURE PRINCIPLE

Every intervention, session, or series of sessions has a beginning, middle, and end.

Closure is achieved when the whole person, in accordance with his or her changing and unchanging limitations, can sustain the changes introduced without further intervention. In order to optimize and stabilize the results of any intervention, session, or series of sessions, the newly emerging pattern of order must be brought to its highest level of integration.

Even though there are patients who seem to require therapy to the end of their life, every therapeutic intervention, every session, and every series of sessions have varying degrees of closure. "More of the same" must eventually give way to another approach (either within one's therapeutic system or to some other system), to ceasing therapy for a period of time, or finally to ceasing therapy altogether.

An Example of Principle-Centered Decision Making

In order to answer the three questions of therapy ("What do I do first, next, and when am I finished?") in accordance with the principles of intervention a thorough examination of the patient is required. Within the context of one's system of intervention, the examination should attempt to locate all the patient's order-thwarters within the five categories of assessment and determine which levels of the whole require enhancement. Before every session or intervention the holistic practitioner should ask:

Which aspects of the whole person—as represented in the five categories of assessment and if properly normalized, organized, and enhanced—will bring the highest level of integration to the whole?

Further evaluation must then determine whether the body can adapt to, support, or has enough continuity and palintonic balance to appropriately respond to and maintain the proposed intervention strategies and tactics. If there is not sufficient adaptability, support, continuity, or palintonicity present, then each one of these conditions of hierarchical order must be established in a sequence of interventions that will both normalize somatic dysfunction and promote the highest level of integration possible for each particular client.

Let us consider a simplified example. Suppose our initial examination of a client with back pain uncovers a complicated array of myofascial and articular fixations in the lumbar and pelvic regions with no radiculopathy. If all the principles are reasonably fulfilled within the client's body, then we can precede directly to treating the areas of myofascial and articular strain. However, such a case is exceedingly rare to the point of being non-existent. Typically, most bodies display a complicated array of imbalances and injuries accompanied by many characteristic and not so characteristic patterns of compensation that run through the entire soma.

Examination most often reveals that some principles are better fulfilled than others and that most bodies require a number of sessions before normalization and enhancement begin to appear. If our imagined client is like most people, back pain is embedded in a structure that displays varying degrees of palintonic imbalance, loss of adaptability, and lack of support and continuity. For example, a patient with an imbalance between the agonist and antagonist muscle groups of the flexors and extensors of the neck and lower back and pelvis displays one kind of palintonic imbalance. Often this lack of back/front balance is displayed by hyper-erect bodies that arch backward when seen from the side. Lack of extensor/flexor balance can also be present in inside/outside imbalance when, for example, the rectus abdominis is stronger than the psoas. Lack of support is often found in bodies where one leg is more valgus and more externally rotated than the other or when the feet are too pronated to support repositioning of a tilted pelvis. Loss of adaptability can be found throughout most bodies. For most people the upper thoracic spine, ribs, shoulder girdle, and sometimes the arms and cranium display a complicated array of myofascial and articular fixations that will not adapt to significant changes in the lower spine and pelvis. For a lesser number of other people the upper quadrant is flexible enough to adapt, but the lower quadrant is so severely restricted that any attempt to introduce change in the pelvic and lumbar region rebounds against fixations in the lower legs and feet even though the legs are providing proper support.

In the initial examination, and continually during the application of techniques, the holistic practitioner must determine how well each principle is fulfilled, which ones are better fulfilled than others, and in what order each one should be fulfilled. If the examination reveals that our client cannot adapt because he or she has fixations in the cranium, cervicals, and in the celomic sacs, or that the body cannot support any of our proposed strategies, or that there are significant back/front imbalances, we must decide the best areas in which to begin our work. Beginning with work on the legs and feet in such a case is usually a mistake. Since work in the lower quadrant inevitably releases upward through the body, two problems would likely arise from such a strategy: 1) the upper quadrant fixations would become more severe by working in the feet and legs, and 2) the upper fixations would keep the lower quadrant from holding its changes. Any attempt to affect back/front balance would also run up against the same sort of difficulties. So the first interventions are most often aimed at the inability of the upper quadrant to adapt. In fact, because of the complicated array of strains that often appear in the thorax, working on the feet and lower legs, as the second session of the formulistic ten series dictates, can be premature.

If a sufficient number of adaptability issues can be handled in the first session, then the next session could deal with either the support or palintonic issues—depending on which one, if properly manipulated, will most benefit the whole person. Depending on the client's body, support may be a more important issue than the palintonic imbalances. Sometimes establishing proper support eases palintonic problems, and sometimes easing palintonic issues creates better support. If the client has excessive spinal curvature, experience has shown that some attention must be devoted to creating adaptability throughout the body especially in the extremities, as well as creating support and back/front balance before such a spine can be properly addressed.

On some occasions we may think that we are ready to address the fixations (order-thwarters) in the lumbar and pelvic regions only to discover that the client was sexually abused as a child and has not resolved these abuse issues. Such a discovery means that any attempt to work on the pelvis will more than likely be met with unconscious resistance. Since the client would be incapable of adapting to our strategy, we would have to postpone the pelvic work until our client had sufficiently resolved these problems, either through our work or the interventions of another therapist. Sometimes our attempts to establish support or palintonic balance create unanticipated strain patterns in other areas of the body or disrupt previously achieved levels of organization. Under such circumstances we must attempt to reestablish them again or in new ways.

If after a number of sessions we determine to the best of our ability that the principles have been sufficiently fulfilled, we can then proceed to work on the pelvis and lumbar region and reasonably expect the client to enjoy some longer-lasting relief from pain. Relieving the pain, however, is not the same as resolving the client's somatic dysfunction or enhancing function through structural integration. More work is usually required in order to achieve the important holistic goal of enhancing the structure and functioning of the whole person. But we should not forget that the goal of structural integration will always be limited by unresolved pain and dysfunction.

Again the holistic practitioner asks, "Which aspects of the whole person if normalized and enhanced will most benefit the organization and functioning of the whole?" Once the area is decided upon by proper examination and evaluation, the practitioner then asks whether the client's body has sufficient adaptability, support, or palintonic balance to maintain the proposed changes and remain stable afterward. If the answer is no to any of the principle questions, the condition specified by the principle in question must be established. As the conditions specified by each principle are established or determined to already be established, the practitioner then proceeds toward establishing the next highest level of order and functioning that the client can handle until the body has achieved the highest level it can. When the whole person has achieved the highest level of integration possible within the constraints of his or her changing and unchanging limitations, more therapy becomes a waste of time and closure is achieved. Therapy ceases and the client's body continues to change and evolve on its own until it meets the next level or levels of fixation that interfere with its development.

Whether a client comes for the relief of pain or for structural integration and the enhancement of function, the decision-making process is the same. Obviously the process can be far more complicated than the above examples demonstrate, often ranging over many more assessment types than the ones discussed. The strategies and tactics as well as the order and depth in which the principles are fulfilled vary from person to person and from session to session depending upon the level and depth of the individual clients' fixations across the five categories of assessment. Strategies and tactics are created and abandoned to suit the needs of each client, but the principles of intervention remain the guiding light in terms of which all of our clinical decisions are made.

CHAPTER 5

Psychobiological Assessment: The Intertwining of Flesh and Thought

A rational, principle-centered decision-making process depends on a number of factors. Besides the obvious need for understanding the principles of intervention, it also requires a highly developed set of assessment skills designed to give practitioners the ability to identify the order-thwarters that are interfering with the client's integration and well-being. I briefly sketched the five types of assessment and intervention in Chapter Two. In this chapter I want to revisit the question of assessment and illustrate by means of examples the nature of the psychobiological type. The adherence to an unhealthy worldview, physical and emotional trauma, confused thought processes, and the like are all examples that fall under the psychobiological assessment category.

Surprisingly, adherence to an unhealthy worldview can have much the same effect as repressed emotions. Psyche and soma are so intertwined that often unless both are released neither will release independently of the other. Two extremes are possible: a person's worldview can be anchored in distortions of the flesh or somatic dysfunctions can be fused to a problematic worldview.

"Wait a minute!" you may be thinking, "Aren't these mental health issues that are beyond the purview of manual therapy and better handled by trained mental health professionals such as psychiatrists, psychotherapists, and counselors?" Generally speaking, they are beyond the scope of the practice of manual therapy, and manual therapy is not a substitute for psychotherapy. But there are times when manual therapy can be very supportive and helpful in the psychotherapeutic process. It is especially helpful when psychological issues are anchored in distortions of the flesh. If these somatic fixations are not recognized or handled properly, they can interfere with the progress of therapy.

For example, it is not uncommon for a manual therapist to be working on an area of the client's body that seems particularly defended against change when all of a sudden the client is flooded with feeling and begins to sob. When sobbing subsides, the restricted area in the client's body easily releases. Because repressed feelings and memories are anchored in the body, holistic manual therapy can be very helpful in releasing them. Otherwise, if they are not handled, therapy could bog down and go nowhere.

The reverse is also common. What is often considered merely a structural (bodily) issue (such as a vertebra that is "out of place" or a pelvis that is tipped anteriorly) can be partially maintained by adherence to an unhealthy worldview. If a manual therapist does not recognize or know how to handle these cognitive fixations, they are likely to impede the client's progress.

One of the signs of a healthy integrated person consists in a high degree of freedom from conflicted ways of thinking. In contrast, the embodiment of a conflicted way of thinking involves more than adopting an unhealthy point of view. It is not uncommon for the body to express distorted ways of thinking by distorting the flesh.

In order to illuminate how the assessment type called psychobiological intentionality (or orientation) figures in designing treatment, we will examine a number of examples. But first, three terminological points are in order. Unfortunately, there is no single word in English for the whole human person that does not anticipate or assume some version of metaphysical dualism where the body is considered just another object that is separate from the mind. "Psychobiological" goes somewhat in the opposite direction and seems to adequately blur the distinction between mind and body. As for the concept of intentionality, it will be discussed in Chapter Six. Finally, as I point out in the Introduction and further explicate in Chapter Two and Chapter Ten, I use the word "order-thwarter" instead of words such as "dysfunctional" or "fixation" because it implies that a pattern of distress lives in relationship, not as an isolated symptom.

With that said, let's return to our discussion of psychobiological assessment. As I've said before, the order in which interventions are made during a session is every bit as important as the interventions. You cannot change the order-thwarters you do not perceive—except by accident. Assessment is a form of highly skilled perception. It takes training and practice to recognize the order-thwarters characteristic of each assessment type and have at your disposal the means to change them.

Example 1: Afraid to Slouch

This example is a straightforward case of how belief in a theory can make you go rigid.

Robert received his Rolfing session as a model in an advanced Rolfing class I co-taught with William (Bill) Smythe, an Advanced Rolfer and a master of trauma work. Robert arrived for his first session complaining of aches and pain and a great deal of strain and overall tightness. He went on to say how the Rolfing he received years ago had freed him from a long-standing depression. Rolfing had allowed his collapsed body to find a more upright stance. But significantly, he held that stance rigidly, maintaining his body in tension-laden conformity to an unyielding notion of ideal posture. Bill correctly perceived that he maintained this hyper-erect posture because he was afraid that he might collapse back into his depression. Over the years this rigid stance had become all but cemented in place causing him a lot of discomfort. He had sought further sessions of Rolfing for relief, but to no avail. Much of the work he received was forceful and painful. Bill immediately recognized the futility of the forceful method and approached the sessions differently. Realizing that some of Robert's rigidity was rooted in a traumatically induced immobility response, Bill masterfully employed very gentle techniques designed to thaw aspects of Robert's soma, which were immobilized in high sympathetic arousal. The strategy worked well and when coupled with a little philosophical counseling about the problematic nature of the concept of an "ideal body" and how his adherence to it was creating his discomfort, Robert was able to finally let go of his rigidity and release some deeply held anguish. As a result, his tension began to disappear and his life became easier.

Example 2: Somatically Maintained Worldview

This example dramatically demonstrates how easing patterns of strain and introducing a higher level of organization in the body and its relation to gravity can profoundly alter one's ethics and worldview. This case is a clear demonstration of how a person's worldview can be somatically maintained.

Beth was in her mid-thirties when she sought my services as a Rolfer. She was extremely intelligent and witty. Since she did not trust men, she was wary of me and shared very little of herself during the early stages of our working together. Only after she gained some trust in me did she tell me that her father was horribly abusive. He often referred to her as a "little piece of shit." She was a single mother of a ten-year-old son. After a number of failed relationships and a very difficult marriage and divorce, she gave up trying to have relationships with men and chose a lesbian lifestyle. She lived with her lesbian lover and worked hard as a waitress trying to make ends meet.

Her body was amazingly immature in its appearance. If you covered her face in her before photographs, she looked like a fearful, disheartened, deflated twelve-year-old. After only a few sessions, however, I noticed some rather dramatic changes. Besides the obvious improvements in posture and the increasing ease of movement that are so characteristic of Rolfing, her body began to mature. She became more animated and her body caught up to her chronological age. Almost overnight she began to look like a mature woman. Her change was so dramatic that all her friends commented on it.

After our third session, she told me that she had stopped shoplifting. Until that moment I had no idea that she engaged in this sort of activity. She shared that she had suddenly realized that she had been projecting her anger at her father and the men in her life onto the rich men she imagined owned these stores. She told me that she only shoplifted at the big department stores. She justified her behavior to herself on the grounds that these men had more money than they needed, that she was owed something for the suffering she had experienced at the hands of all the other rotten men in her life, and that she had a hard time making ends meet.

Three or four sessions after she gave up shoplifting, she told me that she had ended her relationship with her female lover. She acknowledged that she wanted warmth and love in her life just like everybody else. But she also admitted that she had become too frightened to pursue any kind of intimate relationship with men because her experiences with them had been so painful. So she had chosen a lesbian lover instead. Once she realized that she was using homosexual love to satisfy her needs, she realized that she was using her lover in a way that was no longer right for her or fair to her lover.

Before she shared these revelations, Beth and I never talked about shoplifting or her sexuality. She came to these changes in her psychobiological orientation on her own. All I did was work with her body in a respectful way that did not violate her boundaries or contribute to her low self-esteem. If she had asked for my opinion about her shoplifting, I would have discussed the ethics of her behavior as a philosophical counselor. But I also realize in retrospect that any discussion about the ethics of her shoplifting would have been futile. Her shoplifting was fused to her pain and anger at men and bound too severely to her immature and immobile body structure. Even if Beth had brought the topic up for discussion herself, I am convinced that any attempt to address the ethics of her shoplifting would have compelled her to terminate her work with me. I probably would have been perceived as just another self-righteous patriarch telling her what a terrible person she was.

Her immobility and immature appearance were tied to the traumas of her life. She was somewhat dissociated, and her body was frozen in a high state of sympathetic arousal. Like every other severely traumatized individual, she had lost much of her ability to defend herself. Her remarkable transformation during the early stages of our work together began with her being able to trust me and the process of Rolfing. As the Rolfing manipulations eased the patterns of strain in her fascia, she was able to discharge her highly tuned sympathetic state and clarify her self-sensing. As a result, she regained more of the inherent mobility and motility of her body, recovered many of her lost resources, and, as a result, learned to better fend and care for herself. She improved her financial condition by receiving some training and getting a better paying job. As she released her fear and clarified her self-sensing, she learned that she could trust herself and her body to guide her choices toward a more mature future.

This case is particularly interesting because it shows how changes to the organization, motility, and mobility of the soma can profoundly alter a person's worldview. These changes in Beth's psychobiological orientation were the direct result of the myofascial manipulations of Rolfing. Philosophical counseling and any kind of verbal therapy would have been a waste of time. The fact that she experienced Rolfing in a safe therapeutic environment was also a critical factor in her transformation. But it is important to realize that in the early stages of our work together, I did not employ any philosophical or psychotherapeutic techniques.

This case clearly demonstrates the profound hold our flesh can exercise on our ideas and how we live our lives. It also underlines the importance of giving the body its due in any psychotherapeutic and philosophical counseling session. If the flesh does not agree with the logic of a verbal intervention, there may be no significant change in a person's worldview. And, as this case so clearly demonstrates, sometimes all that is required to change a person's outlook on life is a little more order in the flesh and a little more clarity in self-sensing. Of course, it is not always as simple as this case makes it appear, and I am not suggesting that therapists should make it their business to change a person's sexual orientation.

Example Three: Philosophically Maintained Pain

Donna's case is a bit more complicated than Beth's but demonstrates in a fascinating way how a person's tacit worldview can contribute to maintaining her pain. Donna is a married working woman in her late thirties and the mother of two children. She sought out Rolfing for the relief of pain in her right shoulder, which became more pronounced with movement. She received a number of sessions from me and other therapists in our physical therapy clinic where we practiced a team approach based on integrating the three paradigms of practice. The manual therapy she received gave her little to no relief. After a few weeks of therapy at our clinic she went back to her doctor. He discovered that there was a bone spur on her acromion and recommended surgery. After the surgery Donna returned to our clinic for more manual therapy. She experienced no complications from the surgery, and her pain was well on the way to being alleviated. Unfortunately, fate intervened and involved her in an automobile accident. Her pain came back with a vengeance. She continued to receive intensive manual therapy at our clinic for a number of months following her accident. I worked with her at least once a week. After most sessions she would get some relief. But always her pain returned—sometimes within a few hours, sometimes within a day.

At first I didn't notice the almost obsessive way Donna continually complained and worried about her situation. After all, her pain was real and it was seriously interfering with her busy life. She clearly wanted to get well. She was not an overly controlling person or an obsessive compulsive. Like most people whose pain continues well past normal expectations, she often wondered why this had happened to her and was beginning to fear that her shoulder would never heal. Since shoulder injuries and rotator cuff strains are often very difficult to treat and sometimes never get better, her fears were well grounded.

She engaged me in a lot of talking about her situation. We talked about the metaphysical and spiritual implications of pain. We discussed how she held her body in various activities, how she walked, how she sat, and so forth. We also discussed her sleeping position. She mentioned that she slept on her side with her arm above her head. For obvious reasons, I strongly suggested that she not sleep this way. She took my advice and her pain let up just a bit, but not enough to satisfy her or me. During every session she talked and worried more and more about her problem, always trying to come up with a new way to adjust or change the way she did things. Donna always shared her latest strategy for recovery and her worried disappointment in its failed results. Slowly I began to realize that her worry and need to do something about her pain was a bit excessive.

Finally, I suggested that she try an idea. I explained that I had noticed over many years of working with people in pain that the kind of worrying she was engaging in often interfered with healing. I said that excessive reflection on our own suffering was sometimes a serious impediment to recovery. I asked her to imagine a situation in which she was surrounded by all the healing energy she needed to get well and that this healing energy was doing everything it could to get into her body to do its work. "Imagine," I said, "that your excessive dwelling on your suffering is the very thing that is preventing the energy from entering your system, and that what you must do to allow the energy to do its work is to stop worrying." I also asked her to be attentive to how she responded whenever she felt even the slightest twinge of pain, and to notice how easily the appearance of her pain catapulted her once again into dwelling on and worrying about her shoulder. I directed her to set her worrying aside and not to tarry the slightest with her pain when it showed itself.

After two weeks of not dwelling on her shoulder, her pain decreased by ninety percent. She was greatly encouraged by this turn of events. We continued her therapy at the clinic and she continued to improve. Even though she was almost pain free, during a session she began worrying about the small discomfort that she was still feeling in her shoulder. As she talked about the lingering discomfort, her worry escalated and suddenly the severity of her pain increased to the level it had been right after the accident. She was horrified, and I was aghast at how much pain she was experiencing.

I immediately asked her to experience both the fullness of her pain and how it was being held by her in reflection. I asked her to notice how her worrying and reflecting on her situation was sufficient to bring her pain back. I suggested that she cease her worrying. She complied and as she gave up her reflective worry, her pain dissipated just as quickly as it appeared. We decided that the appearance of her pain at this point in her therapy could be used as a sign of her excessive reflection. From that moment on whenever she felt pain she simply stopped thinking about it and it disappeared.

She continued the team approach at our clinic and was happy with the results. A few weeks later I saw her for another session. Her pain was negligible, and she was confident that her life was back to normal. We chatted easily as I worked with her shoulder. She reported that she was very upset at the news that Linda McCartney, wife of ex-Beatle, Paul McCartney, had died of cancer. I was surprised by this and asked why the death of someone she only read about would be so upsetting to her. She replied that Linda McCartney was a vegetarian, that she practiced yoga, and had worked hard at living a healthy peaceful life. Donna also devoted herself to a similar program and confessed that it was unnerving to learn that someone could die of cancer even after devoting so much of herself toward living a healthy life.

Curious, I asked her if she believed something like the following: there are a set of rules that define how life is to be lived, and that if we do our best to discover and follow them, God or the universe will make sure nothing too awful befalls us. Immediately the intense pain in her shoulder reappeared and her eyes filled with tears. As further investigation and discussion revealed, even though she had never really brought her view into full reflective awareness, she tacitly held a view something like the one I articulated for her. As it turned out, this view was at the heart of her excessive attempts to control and deal with her pain. She believed that if she could only discover how she had strayed from the right way of living and using her body, she could correct her mistakes and be free of her difficulties.

We talked in some detail about her tacit presupposition. I did not try to argue against her view, but only gave her other views against which she could contrast her pre-reflective tacit worldview. I explained how other spiritual traditions left lots of room for the occurrence of random, meaningless events that are capable of derailing one's life. I also mentioned that some traditions even believed that God was also learning and evolving. Once she brought her tacit worldview into reflective awareness and was able to contrast it with other views, she realized that she really was not committed to her view and abandoned it on the spot. She has been free of shoulder pain ever since.

I was surprised by how quickly and easily Donna's pain disappeared upon giving up her excessive reflection and worry. I was even more surprised by how suddenly it returned when she re-engaged her excessive worry. But it wasn't until she shared her upset over Linda McCartney's death that I realized that her excessive worry was rooted in a tacit philosophical view of how the world worked, a view that unreflectively spurred her to continually interrogate her pain and experiment with ways to manage it. She was an intelligent woman who had her life in good order. She was not driven by a neurotic need to control her world, and she was not an obsessive compulsive. But her unexamined worldview, which may have been influenced by her Catholic upbringing, drove her to take too much responsibility for healing herself and compelled her to think excessively about her problem and how to solve it. You might say she had a bad case of philosophically maintained pain. Clearly, if I had pursued manual therapy in a purely structural/functional way and had never uncovered her tacit worldview, Donna would still be in pain today.

These three examples are meant to illustrate how the psychobiological intentionality assessment type comes into play. Placing this kind of emphasis upon the psychobiological intentionality assessment type should not imply that the other assessment types are not relevant. Further assessment would show that all three of the clients needed varying degrees of structural and functional work. Since an order-thwarter in one assessment type usually shows up more or less as an order-thwarter in all, you should come to expect that you almost always work with a number of assessment types and their ways of intervening at one and the same time. Our fourth example is an actual assessment designed to demonstrate how all the assessment types can be relevant to designing a session.

Example 4: Immaculate Perception

This last example is based on a simplified version of an actual assessment. Its purpose is to demonstrate the depth and kind of perception that is really possible and available to us. But you will not learn how to perform this uncanny way of perceiving until we get to Chapter Seven where I present the simple three-step method I created to train practitioners. For now, simply appreciate the way this example displays how a complex pattern of order-thwarters reveals itself in relation to the whole across all the categories of assessment to an experienced practitioner. It demonstrates the process a practitioner might go through in order to perceive at this level of sophistication.

Imagine that you are about to begin assessing a client with back pain. If you are a Rolfer, you might begin your session with a visual inspection of your client in order to evaluate how well she appropriates gravity. Your training and years of experience in geometric, structural, functional, energetic, and psychobiological assessment have given you the perceptual skills necessary to make this kind of assessment. You notice that she has many of the key characteristics of the structural type Jan Sultan called "externally rotated": high stiff arches, externally rotated femurs, posteriorly tipped pelvis, diminished A-P spinal curvature, a relatively flat occiput, etc. As you continue your assessment, you notice that she doesn't have clear centerline, her pelvis is right rotated, her sacrum is bilaterally fixed posteriorly, and there is strain in the left, abdominal region. As you assess her psychobiological orientation, you sense that she is grounded, and that she comports herself with confidence and ease. At the same time, you feel a sense of withdrawal and sadness in her chest. Then you notice that she is tired at the same time you feel that her cranium is in trouble.

In order to bring the information gleaned from your assessment to a more full-bodied perception of her living form, you shift your orientation from actively looking at patterns to getting out of the way and letting your client's body show you its problems. As she lies supine on your table, you gently place your hands on her head using your favorite vault hold and just wait. Your job, at this point, is not to have a job. You wait and do nothing. You are no longer actively trying to assess your client's structure, function, energy, or psychobiological intentionality. You don't even think about trying to change her for the better. Instead, you shift your orientation from trying to accomplish results and evaluating structure to an orientation of allowing what is to show itself. You simply get out of the way by expanding your perceptual field, dropping your self, and opening a loving space.

The clarity and safety of this clearing makes it possible for the being of your client to wordlessly reveal her troubles to you. As you continue to create this loving space, you often close your eyes as a way to see more clearly and to encourage more and more aspects of your client's problems to show themselves to you. In order to further expand and deepen your perception, you take your hands off your client's head and feel-perceive her whole body and energy field with your whole body and energy field. After a time, a perspective begins to come into focus and you finally get your first glimpse of a unified pattern of distortion and its relation to the whole: you perceive a cranial shutdown, the lack of a clear center line, a bulging out of the energy field around the lower left region of the abdomen coupled with feelings of sadness and anger saturating an intensely held strain in the peritoneal sac around the descending colon; you more clearly perceive her posterior sacrum and the rotation of her entire pelvis to the right. As often happens, when your eyes are closed, your mind starts to drift as if you were in the first stages of sleep. Suddenly, a compelling image of your client being traumatized appears and with the image comes the conviction that she was ten years old when the incident occurred.

Notice how all the information you gleaned finally congealed into a unified perception of her structural, functional, energetic, and psychobiological way of being. In the beginning of your assessment you were actively engaged in the process of evaluation. Much of the information you gathered about your client was the direct result of actively engaging and searching for patterns and structural imbalance. Recall how you saw that your client was an external type, for example. Before you learned the internal/external typology, you probably would have noticed how the pelvis was too posterior, how the lumbar and thoracic spines were too flat, how the legs were valgus, and so on. But you wouldn't have grasped the significance of what you saw for the whole structure. You probably would have seen these aspects as individual structural curiosities. You wouldn't have understood that what you were seeing was an expression of the morphological type known as the external type. But now when you look at your client, you immediately and clearly see that she is an external type. As a result, you understand the complicated array of strain patterns with which she struggles in relation to her morphological imperative.

You also began to perceive aspects of her psychobiological intentionality by means of feeling. You felt and saw the confidence in her comportment, while at the same time, sensing her withdrawal, sadness, anger, tiredness, as well as the effect of these aspects on her cranium. This kind of *feeling* in which you perceive the emotional meaning of a person's bearing and structure requires not just the integration of the sensory and the cognitive but also the integration of your feeling-nature. When you can feel aspects as well as see them, your ability to read your client's emotional and psychobiological orientation is much more accurate than when you deduce them from visual patterns displayed by your client's body.

As you continue, you rely less on your senses and more on your feeling-nature to perceive what was going on with your client. Much of the same information appeared, but more of it came to you through your feelings. There is no question, much of what you perceive as a holistic practitioner comes from your senses—but not all. Notice that you can see without your eyes and feel without your hands. You often closed your eyes in order to perceive more clearly, for example. Since you felt what is happening in the lower abdomen and pelvis while your hands were on your client's cranium, you were not feeling with your hands alone. Add to these considerations that you can feel more by not touching your client, and it is clear that you are not perceiving with your senses only—you are also perceiving with your feeling-nature. When you perceive your client's structural problems and her comportment as sad and angry, you are see-feeling by means of the integration of your cognitive, sensory, and feeling-nature.

Let's look more closely at what we actually experience when we perceive with our feeling-nature. Whether you touch your client or remove your hands from her body, when you allow what is to show itself, you often feel in your own body where the problems are in your client's body. Where your client has a problem in her body, typically, you feel a kind of pressure or fullness in the same place in your body. As you continue to attend to what is showing itself to you, the vague sense of pressure begins to come into focus and you begin to see-feel it as an emotional, energetic, and structural distortion in the descending colon that affects the pelvis and right knee. If you close your eyes, you may also notice that you also see in your mind's eye the same pattern of distortion.

The more anatomy and physiology you know, the more you perceive in your client, especially if you keep an open heart. The better you know anatomy and the freer you are of emotional fixations and conflicts, the better you are able to perceive the details of what is being shown to you. In this example, if you didn't know the anatomy of the organs, the vague sense of pressure would remain a vague sense of pressure indicating a problem somewhere in the left lower region of the abdomen. But since you do know the anatomy of this region of the body, you see-feel the detail that indicates an organ.

It is as if your energy field and your feeling-nature overlap. You not only feel with your whole body, you also feel with your energy field. You feel in your own energy field the place where your client's energy is distorted. The more familiar you become with the energy patterns that are part of your clients' problems, the more clearly you feel them.

There is an important difference between perceiving with your eyes and perceiving with your feeling-nature. When you perceived your client as an external morphological type, you perceived her as other than yourself and "over there." When you felt your client's structural, energetic, and emotional difficulties, you felt all of these aspects as "over here" and in yourself. There was next to no distance between you and these aspects of your client. You felt them as if they were your own, because your way of knowing them is by feeling them in yourself and because feeling-perception is non-dualistic, participatory, and not based on reflective thinking.

If you continue to allow what is to show itself, the whole pattern of distortion and its relationship to the whole comes into clearer focus and you see-visualize-feel it as a unified gestalt. Since your client has emotional issues, you feel her anger or sadness in yourself and it will saturate your perception of and be a part of the unified gestalt. The unified gestalt that constitutes your perception of your client is the result of integrating cognition with your senses and feeling-nature. At one and the same time, you are one with her condition because you feel it and separate from her condition because she is not you. Simultaneously, you feel your client's distortions in yourself and see them in her body. Your perception of your client's condition is not a matter of having two different perceptions, one in yourself and one of her "over there." Rather, your perception is one integrated unified gestalt in which you are both one with your client and separate from your client.

So far we have only scratched the surface of our feeling-nature, and we still don't know what part of our anatomy or mind is responsible for this kind of perception. We perceive a rose with our eyes, hear a sound with our ears, smell an odor with our nose, relish an apple with our sense of taste, and feel a rough edge with our sense of touch. But with what sense or senses do we perceive a client's energy and emotional patterns, thwarts to wholeness, or that something is amiss? Whatever this perceptual system is, it consists of the integration of our senses, cognition, feeling-nature, and energetic field. While it is clear that it must involve the brain and nervous system (the senses) as well as what we call mind, it is also clear that it surpasses these systems. Unlike our eyes and ears, it has no specific location. We are driven to the conclusion that this perceptual system is none other than our body-mind and the field around it. For want of a better term, we can call it the *somatic field*.

Conclusion: Where Is the Human Sensorium?

If asked where the seat of perception is or which system is responsible for perception, without much hesitation most people would probably answer that the sensorium is the brain and nervous system. For humans and other vertebrates, this answer seems like a reasonable one. But our excursion into feeling led us to the startling conclusion that our perceptual abilities are greater and more expansive than we suspected. They encompass not only our feeling-nature and whole body, including the brain and nervous system, but also extend into the field around our bodies. If this observation is correct, we must also conclude that the human sensorium is the somatic field.

Our feeling-nature is not only deeply intertwined with and embedded in all our states of awareness; it is also what we share with all living creatures. It is how other forms of life, especially those without a brain or nervous system, perceive their world. Furthermore, what we recognize in ourselves as consciousness is a highly evolved elaboration of the same feeling-nature that all life shares.

Our feeling-nature is a non-dualistic, participatory way of knowing that is not founded in reflective thinking. It permeates every dimension of our being and every level of awareness and is fully integrated with our sensory and cognitive nature. Even though we regularly take no notice of it because our consciousness is dominated by our reflective "I-am-self," it is always there bringing us into unity with our surroundings and revealing the greater ocean of sentience of which we are a part.

Two extremes emerged from our discussion and we saw how a person's worldview can be rooted in her soma in one case, and, in the other, how a person's worldview can contribute to maintaining her pain. The first you could say is an example of a somatically maintained worldview and the second an illustration of philosophically maintained pain. The example of being afraid to slouch is a more straightforward example. It illustrates how adherence to a theory motivated by fear can over time all but cement in place a rigid way of being. I picked these four examples to illustrate the relevance and workings of the assessment types with special emphasis on the psychobiological. Since the usual way we assess clients would not emphasize just one type, the fourth example shows how a creative and experienced holistic somatic practitioner might work with all of the assessment types. But I also wanted all of these examples to suggest the intertwining of psyche and soma, and how difficult in practice it is to separate our nature into two separate and distinct categories of mind and body. At this point in our investigation these comments are only meant to be suggestive. I am just sowing the seeds for deconstructing metaphysical dualism in Chapter Eight. We will return to the nature of perception and its philosophical underpinnings in Chapter Six and present the three-step method for training perception in Chapter Seven.

CHAPTER 6

Seeing

There are many forms of assessment available to holistic somatic practitioners. Some are easy and straightforward and don't demand much skill to perform. For example, you might time how long it takes for a client to get up from a chair, walk to another chair, and sit. Or you might measure range of motion. Some forms of assessment require training and much higher levels of skill to perform accurately. Chapter Five provided us with quite a number of assessments based on highly developed perceptual skills. For example, we said of the client discussed in example 4 that she was grounded and comported herself with confidence but also showed a sense of withdrawal and sadness in her chest. We also noted that she may have been traumatized when she was ten years old. We discussed feeling order-thwarters in the pelvis and sacrum by cradling her head in the practitioner's hands. We mentioned perceiving energy distortions in and around her body.

We usually don't question how we know the easy straightforward assessments are correct, because they tend to be clearly based on objective grounds. But with respect to the other kinds of assessments mentioned above, we tend to be suspicious of them because they seem too subjective to compel assent. What we will discover as we engage in this investigation of subjectivity and objectivity is that the so-called subjective assessments are akin to aesthetic judgments. By Chapter Ten it will be clear why holistic assessments and aesthetic experience are neither subjective nor objective.

Clearly, skillful perception is central to the practice of holistic manual therapy. Without it, therapy would be analogous to a blind cat sometimes catching a dead mouse. It also may very well be the most difficult skill to teach holistic practitioners. Anybody who knows anything about Rolf knows that she was possessed of an uncanny perceptual ability. She was known to have said to her students that they were only *looking* when they needed to be *seeing*. Most of us probably have an intuitive sense of what she was driving at with this distinction. But, when we try to make her meaning fully explicit, words escape us. To this day, there is no agreed-upon standard way of understanding what "seeing" consists of or how to teach it.

The purpose of this chapter and the next is to remedy this difficulty by examining the philosophical presuppositions that stand in our way and articulating a simple self-teaching three-step exercise in *seeing*. I excavated this three-step process from phenomenology and most importantly from Goethe's discovery of "exact sensorial imagination." Throughout this discussion of perception, I relied heavily on both approaches and on Henri Bortoft's way of articulating these two approaches.* Mixed in throughout are my explanations and ruminations. There are probably many reasons behind our difficulties surrounding seeing. One of the most insidious and difficult stumbling blocks comes directly from the influence of René Descartes (1596–1650).

Descartes is rightly regarded as the father of modern philosophy. His philosophy profoundly shaped our world. His influence is so pervasive that even those who have never heard of Descartes have adopted his framework. His philosophy attempted to lay the rational foundations of science. As a result, his efforts inaugurated our modern scientific age. He reconfigured the content of the subject/object distinction so drastically and narrowly that all interaction between them was rendered utterly impossible. How we think about perception is deeply informed by Descartes's self-defeating, overly narrow comprehension of subjectivity and objectivity. At times you can even find Descartes's philosophy

---

*See Bortoft's two books on phenomenology and Goethe's science of quality: *Taking Appearances Seriously: The Dynamic Way of Seeing in Goethe and European Thought* (Edinburgh: Floris Books, 2012); *The Wholeness of Nature: Goethe's Way toward a Science of Conscious Participation in Nature* (New York: Lindisfarna Press, 1996).

lurking in the shadows of explanations by cognitive scientists who reject Descartes's philosophy.

Before we can properly explore the contours of perception and vindicate the function of holistic assessments, we need to expose how the Cartesian worldview undermines every attempt to understand the phenomena in question.

Cartesian Worldview

Pictured here is a cartoon summary of the *causal/representational theory of perception*. Many problematic presuppositions find their source in the confusion surrounding this widely accepted theory, first championed by Descartes and Galileo (1564–1642). On this view, knowledge of the external world comes about through the way our senses and nervous system causally interact with material reality outside of us. From the interaction of our senses with physical reality, our brain produces ideas that serve as representations (mental pictures) of whatever is beyond our senses. According to the theory, we do not have direct access to the world external to us. We only have access to the appearances, that is, to the representational ideas in our mind.

The theory is supposed to explain how we have knowledge of the external world. Unfortunately, the theory makes the very thing it seeks to explain impossible. In order for us to know whether an idea is a hallucination cooked up by the brain or a true representation, we must be able to compare the idea with the object represented. Comparing idea and object is only possible if we have access to both idea and object. But the theory rules out this possibility. It clearly states that we only have access to the ideas, not to the

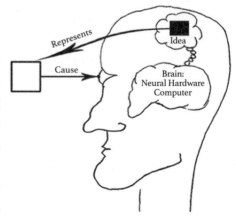

objects themselves. As a result, knowledge of the external world and other minds is impossible on this view.

These problems result from conflating the report of an experience with a causal explanation of the experience. Since a causal explanation can only give us the conditions that make perception possible, it cannot describe our experience. For example, it cannot tell us what the content of our perception is. It cannot tell us what we are seeing. Not only that, the conditions it specifies are, for the most part, a series of causally linked neurological processes that, in principle, cannot be directly experienced. It both mis-describes and conflates the process by which something comes to be seen (comes into appearance) with the object it comes to be seen as (say, a tree). It does not describe our experience of how something comes to be perceived as something. The causal account is not and cannot be a description of our experience because it deals with causally linked neurological processes that can never be our direct experience. To say it differently, you cannot reduce a first-person ontology to a third-person ontology. Clearly, neither the causal nor the representational aspects of the theory are capable of grasping our experiential reality. As we shall see again and again, the causal/representational theory is problematic because it is self-defeating, conflates a causal explanation with a description of experience, and confuses abstract, reflective thought for direct lived experience.

Conflating the report of an experience with an explanation of experience is so pervasive that hardly anyone recognizes the mistake. From the proverbial man in the street to the highly trained neuroscientist, you will see the ever present influence of Descartes's worldview on our thinking.

What we might call Descartes's incommensurability thesis characterizes mind and matter as two opposing incommensurable ontological kinds. Descartes so severely narrowed both sides of the distinction that he forged an unbridgeable gap between them. If you begin, as Descartes does, with the assumption that the body and mind are utterly incommensurable ontological kinds, any interaction between mind and body would be impossible. After all, how can something that takes up no space (mind) affect something that does (body)?

Since the only source of self-activity that this way of thinking recognizes is the human mind, nature and the material world are conceived as inert. The body is part of nature and just as inert. Hence, both nature and body are essentially dead. If the body were truly inert, it would be wholly external to the mind, and it would be experienced as a totally alien object to which we are mysteriously attached. The more you think about this view the more bizarre it seems. If something that takes up no space could not affect something that does, we could not even experience our bodies in the first place.[17]

One of the more pervasive presuppositions of the Cartesian framework is that what is real and objective is what can be measured (e.g., weight, size, shape). The idea that only the measurable is real began with Galileo's methodological recommendation that science investigate only what can be measured. From this methodological recommendation for the conduct of science Galileo drew the unwarranted metaphysical conclusion that only what can be measured is real. Quite apart from the metaphysical conclusion not following from the methodological recommendation, this claim is suspect for other reasons. For example, if only what is measurable is real, what are we to think of the act of measurement itself? Can it be measured?

The incommensurability thesis claims that physical objects take up space and are subject to time. Mental events are temporal but do not occupy space. The whole of the physical universe is a mechanical event composed of mechanical events. Whatever cannot be measured, such as the sweetness of strawberries or the redness of apples is subjective. Our bodies are nothing more than soft machines inhabited by a ghostlike phenomenon we call consciousness. The subject side is the mind, the in-here, the enclosed thinking self. It is private, isolated, closed off, and separate from the material world, and ontologically separate and distinct from the body. The object side is seen as the measurable, mechanical, non-conscious out-there. It is useful to ask: do you really experience yourself as an enclosed, non-spatial in-here mysteriously relating through a soft-machine body to a non-conscious, mechanical out-there?

Clearly, Descartes's way of articulating the difference between mind and body makes their interaction impossible. The same considerations demonstrate the impossibility of any interaction between our minds and the external world. How could mechanical processes cause the appearance of representational ideas that don't occupy space? In the end, the concept of an external world is an abstract construct created by the causal theory of perception. No such thing as the external world exists. The concept of an external world is a fiction, a concept that has no referent.

As long as we are under the spell of Descartes's way of distinguishing the mental and physical, we will never be able to make sense of the interaction of mind and body or escape the solipsistic corner into which Descartes painted himself and our culture. The only way out is to start over. As Merleau-Ponty clearly understood, we must replace Descartes's way of understanding mind and matter with a description that captures how mind is unintelligible without body and how mind and body partake of the same reality. In addition to Merleau-Ponty's suggestion to replace Descartes's description, I would also add the idea that mind and body are not two opposed *substances or things*, but two expressions of the *same interdependent activity*. We will return to these issues in the later chapters of this book.

Phenomenology to the Rescue

Key figures in advancing phenomenology are Franz Brentano (discovered intentionality; 1838–1917), Edmund Husserl (considered the father of phenomenology; 1859–1938), Martin Heidegger (championed an existential, hermeneutical phenomenology; 1889–1976), Maurice Merleau-Ponty (extended existential hermeneutical phenomenology to include the lived body and a deeper understanding of perception; 1908–1961), and, of course, Johann Wolfgang von Goethe (practiced a kind of proto-phenomenology and developed a science of quality; 1749–1832).

Phenomenology turns the tables on the Cartesian worldview by embracing experience as it is lived and not as it is thought about later in reflection. Lived experience is experience as we pre-reflectively live through it. The minute we think about what we are doing, we are no longer in the pre-reflective orientation of consciousness. In reflection, the world is experienced as subject and object.

There is plenty of theory associated with phenomenology, but it is more a method for how to attend to experience than a theory of experience. In order to get our bearings, we can begin with a very simple description of how phenomenology approaches perception. Phenomenology begins with the lived experience of perception and attempts to catch the pre-reflective activity of perceiving and the coming into being of its object, as it is occurring. By recognizing the difference between reflection and pre-reflection (lived experience) and staying with the ongoing interplay of reflection and pre-reflection, the phenomenologist participates with what is in the process of appearing or coming to be seen. Implicitly, reflection is always at work making explicit what is only latent in pre-reflective experience. By cultivating this kind of disciplined attentiveness to how things come into being, the phenomenologist is not seduced into substituting abstract theory for lived experience. The phenomenologist is thus able to give descriptions of experience that have not lost touch with the phenomena being investigated.

To catch perception in the act Bortoft says, "there has to be a refocusing of attention from what is conceived to the act of conceiving, *while engaged in the act of conceiving that which is conceived.*"[18] Within experience we must learn to shift our attention away from the achievement of what is experienced to the experience of achieving what is experienced. This shift within consciousness leads to a transformation of our way of seeing that in turn transforms what is seen without adding to its content. We suddenly see in a new way and see what is seen in a new way. This shift is at the heart of seeing and an important part of the first step in learning to see.

Seeing-As and the Shift in Orientation

Let's look at an example of suddenly seeing in a new way. It will be easier to catch the lived activity of perceiving and the required shift in orientation if we use a simple example. Get ready, you are about to catch perception in the act. Redirect your attention to the activity by which a figure emerges from an apparently random bunch of squiggles. When you look at this drawing from Bortoft,[19] what do you see? At first, probably nothing more than a circle with a bunch of meaningless ink splotches. But now look for a giraffe and watch it come into being. Did you suddenly see a giraffe emerge from the splotches? No lines were added to the drawing, nothing about it changed. What changed was that you acquired the appropriate concept of *giraffe*. Once given the concept, you were able to see the giraffe—you were able to call it forth and make what was indeterminate determinate. But notice it was not there in advance of your seeing it. All of this adds up to recognition that perception has a cognitive dimension and whatever we perceive is always perceived "*as* something." We see this as a chair, that as a bird, that as a herd of cows, or that as finding your line, and so forth.

As long as we continue to orient toward nature as an onlooker, in the way the Cartesian philosophy demands, we will remain blind to the intimate intertwining of nature and human nature that is required by this kind of participatory, cognitively infused perception. Not surprisingly, we are brought once more to the inability of the Cartesian subject/object distinction to grasp lived perception. These considerations also demonstrate that to perceive something as something is already the same as perceiving meaning. This conclusion is significant because it also brings us face to face with one of the most important concepts of phenomenology—intentionality.

Intentionality

"The question about intentionality is at bottom a question about meaning. To speak of an intentional act is to speak of an act which reaches toward or gropes for a meaningful content."[20] With the discovery of intentionality and its vectoral character, Husserl was able to transform and reconfigure the simple subject/object distinction into an invariant fundamental condition of experience that limits and makes possible what appears to us. As a result, he was able to begin the process of breaking the stranglehold Cartesian metaphysics had on how we understand our world.

Consider any experience you might have and you will notice that it always has two correlated poles: what is experienced and the manner in which it is experienced. Notice too that what is experienced always involves a figure and a background. Often intentionality is described as the view that experience is always the experience of something. This characterization is not quite adequate because it does not fully grasp how these two poles are always correlated and, hence, mutually implicate each other. Every experiencing is directed toward what is experienced, and everything experienced reflects or refers back to a mode of experiencing. In other words, whenever there is an experience (e.g., an act of perceiving), there is also that which is experienced (e.g., what is perceived). Wherever there is that which is experienced there is a mode of experiencing it. Because they are correlates, they mutually implicate each other. Unlike subject and object, which are late arrivals to the scene, they are not separate and independent. Their relationship is a correlative unity such that one cannot occur without the other, and one cannot be understood or investigated without including the other. This correlative unity is the prior condition of the separation into subject and object. Husserl calls these two correlates "noesis" (the how of appearing) and "noema" (what appears).

When we engage the world cognitively, we step out of the flow of lived experience and become an onlooker/observer standing over and above and separate from what is being seen. You, the seer are the subject, and that which is seen is the object. The object of perception and the subject who perceives it arise together at the same time the subject sees the object as a tree. Subject and object are based upon and emerge from noesis and noema. At this level of analysis, there is no problem with the subject/object distinction.

The problem arises when we mistakenly take that which appears at the reflective level for the process of coming into appearance from the pre-reflective level. Confusing what is seen with the activity of becoming seen is at the heart of the Cartesian worldview and the causal theory of perception. Within the Cartesian framework, seer and seen are viewed as two separate independent aspects of reality in a contingent relationship. If this contingent relationship of subject and object is mistakenly projected onto lived experience, we lose sight of the necessary inseparability of noesis and noema.

If we pay attention and try to catch perception in the act, we will notice that, while there is a distinction between noesis and noema, there is no separation between them. The appearance of the separation only occurs when we focus on what is seen instead of the activity of coming to be seen.

Intentionality is both directed toward the world and solicited by it. Thus, we see that intentionality is also a vectoral structure probing for the emergence of meaningful content. Contrary to Descartes's picture, the discovery of intentionality reveals that consciousness is intrinsically open to the world. Thus, "...far from being self-enclosed, the very nature of consciousness is such that the world is already included within it."[21]

Defining Phenomenology

We can define phenomenology as the art, philosophy, and science of describing what shows itself to us, as it shows itself, without imposing on it any inappropriate conceptual framework and before we turn it into an abstraction. As a way to deepen our understanding of phenomenology, recognize that the word *phenomenon* means *that which shows itself or that which appears*. Accordingly, Heidegger says to do phenomenology is "*to let what shows itself be seen from itself, just as it shows itself from itself*."[22] Bortoft also makes the point that phenomenon means *the showing of what shows itself* or the appearing *of what appears*. Thus, examining the word *phenomenon* brings to light two important aspects of appearing—what appears and the *appearing* of what appears. Another way to make this point is to say that *perception involves both the process by which something comes to be seen (appearing) and the object it comes to be seen as (what appears).* Typically, when we reflect on what is happening, we tend to only pay attention to what appears as an object of perception and miss entirely the process by which it comes into appearance.

Because we have not trained ourselves to pre-reflectively participate with what we are seeing, when something is coming into appearance as something, we pass over its activity of appearing. We miss entirely the activity by which something comes into appearance as something. Comfortable in our reflective stance toward the things of our world, we tend to see only the result of the activity of appearing. If we are seeing something new for the first time, it is easier to participate in its coming into being. Typically, however, we usually focus only on the object of perception and let the lived experience of the appearing itself slip through our fingers. Over time, as we get used to its presence, it eventually recedes into the background, as so much wallpaper.

The *Logos* in phenomenology means *the site at which being (that which shows itself) reveals itself.* Following Bortoft, it would be more precise to say that the Logos is the site at which the *showing* of what shows itself is revealed. Or the Logos is the site at which the appearing of what appears is revealed.

At this point, an important question needs to be asked: "Is it possible to experience what shows itself as it truly shows itself without contaminating your experience of it with your own biases?" Heidegger holds that "Logos" does not mean "the study of," "logic," or "the word," but rather "the site at which being reveals itself." To simplify the history of phenomenology a bit, unlike the early Husserl, Heidegger insisted you can never take a God-like survey of any phenomenon. Because the experience of what shows itself always takes place within its own unique context, you can never give a pure non-contextual description of anything. You can only interpret it. To try to describe a phenomenon without its context is not to experience it as it shows itself. Part of the discipline of phenomenology consists in laying bare the presuppositions and biases that are embedded in the contextualized field in which we always find ourselves. To do phenomenology is to pre-reflectively let what is show itself as it shows itself contextually, and then to appropriately interpret it reflectively.

The practitioner of phenomenology must develop the ability to pre-reflectively experience and feel, without conflict, into what is. In so doing, the practitioner opens an unconflicted space, a clearing, within which the things and people of our world are revealed. By letting this way of seeing be shaped by the phenomena under consideration, reflective interpretations of phenomenology come to rest upon an understanding that participates with what is understood. Phenomenology invites us to remain true to the things themselves and to our experience. Let's accept that invitation and look at how phenomenology advances our understanding of perception and, in particular, how it can illuminate and deepen our understanding of the way of seeing.

Seeing Holistically and the Shift in Orientation

Senior Advanced Rolfing Instructor Jan Sultan's brilliant discovery of the internal/external typology is an excellent example of seeing holistically. It clearly demonstrates the shift in orientation that brings about a new way of seeing things. One day as he was contemplating the craniosacral rhythm, he was taken with how the body went into external and internal rotation. And then it hit him: there are actually two types of bodies in terms of which we can understand how all these structural differences belong together as expressions of a larger unified whole! Before Sultan saw this distinction, no one understood the hidden dynamics of what we were seeing. The whole thing was basically invisible to us. We knew about internally rotated femurs, flat lumbars, high arches, etc., but nobody saw how these patterns fit together to form a whole body pattern. No one saw, for example, that flat lumbars went with externally rotated femurs. Instead, we saw all these odd structural features in a piecemeal fashion. Nobody saw how the human body could be expressed in two coherent patterns. No one saw how all of these different structural features belonged together as a unified relational whole. No one was *seeing* holistically. Knowledge of the craniosacral rhythm had been around for quite a while, but no one saw in it what Sultan saw. I speculate that it took a Rolfer to see two body types. Why? Because Rolfers are always engaged in seeing the whole body even if they are focused on a torsioned sacrum.

Once the distinction was made, everyone could see it. But, like all such discoveries, it seemed too obvious. But prior to Sultan's discovery the typology was actually invisible to us. By making the distinction Sultan made the difference visible for the first time. He did not apply labels to already known objects. His process of discovery brought the typology into being for the very first time. If you look at what he accomplished at the level of subject and object, you will think that the two types were just lying there waiting to be seen. But in point of fact, by making this distinction, Sultan brought them into being so that they could be seen by us in the first place. Thinking the types were "out there" ready to be discovered presupposes that this distinction had already been made.

Sultan's typology came into being the same way the giraffe came into being. At the moment he got the concept and saw the two types, they stood out for the first time—they came into being for the first time. You could also say that they come into meaning. Coming into being or meaning does not imply that there are pre-given things existing "out there" just waiting to be labeled or that what comes into appearance is something we subjectively create.

Coming into being is neither subjective nor objective. We neither create a subjective reality nor discover an objective reality. Rather, it is a matter of "the world 'calling forth' something in me that in turn 'calls forth' something in the world."[23] In part, that means we are led by the power of the thing to manifest itself. We make something stand out, make what was indeterminate determinate—in a word, we *there* it. Because of this calling forth we now see bodies as two kinds, as both related and different at the same time. Speaking holistically, we can say they are related because what is distinguished must be distinguished from something, and that something must be related to what is distinguished. Speaking analytically, they are different because they are distinguishable.

To avoid possible confusion, it might be useful to remind ourselves of the difference between a phenomenological and scientific approach. Claiming, for example, that the body is an assemblage of parts, or a liquid crystalline structure, or a system of movement are all ways of objectifying the body. Obviously, some objectifications are more accurate or useful than others. But ultimately the lived reality of the body, which includes our I-am-self, is the source for all these different views. No objectification can grasp all of what we are moment to moment. But using mathematics to objectify and explain the body is a powerful way to gain understanding.

In contrast, describing the reality of how we live and experience our body-self is part of what phenomenology does. It is important to keep in mind that phenomenology offers not an alternative explanation of the body, but an alternative to explanation. The descriptions of phenomenology are not offered as explanations (in the technical sense), but as ways to understand our lived corporeality. If phenomenology attempts to explain the body, it oversteps its boundaries. Likewise, science oversteps its boundaries when it claims that all other approaches are merely subjective and only the measurable objects of science are real. We met this mistake in Galileo's thinking where he thought that the methodological use of mathematics demanded by science justified his claim that only what is measurable is real. In making such claims, science ceases to be science and transforms itself into bad metaphysics. As long as we recognize that scientific explanations are a particular kind of objectification and understanding that involves measurement, there is no confusion. Only when science tries to tell us what's real and what is merely subjective does it cease to be science and become scientism or bad metaphysics.

In the next chapter we will put these concepts to work and see what we can see.

CHAPTER 7

The Beauty of Normality

Your ability to see beauty in a work of art and integration appear in your client depends on similar conditions. Whether you are appreciating a work of art or the appearance of integration in a client, each in its own way brings with it a deeply felt sense of order and belonging. To appreciate this way of seeing, let's listen to what Rolf herself had to say about perception. Be aware that perception is not limited to the visual. Notice she sometimes recommends that you change your way of being when you work. Shifting your orientation is the first step in learning how to see.

"And when you see normal structure all of a sudden you say, Why yes, of course, I recognize this as normal structure. Oddly enough, we all have intuitive appreciation of the normal. When we see something that is normal we say, Isn't that beautiful?, Doesn't he move beautifully? etc., etc. Nobody asks you to define that beauty, everybody recognizes it. It's an intuitive appreciation of normalcy."[24] With this insight, we have arrived at what the goal of integrating the body in gravity looks like before it becomes an abstraction. The claim that beauty is the intuitive appreciation of normalcy shows us how indicators of order, such as structural integration and functional economy, were experienced before they became abstractions. Even though the beauty of normalcy cannot be captured by the narrowly conceived categories of subjectivity and objectivity, it is as much a part of our reality as a stone is. Moreover, if anything is a clear and certain indicator that a holistic session is over, the appearance of beauty is certainly one of the more profound.

The Opposite of Aesthetic Is Anesthetic

Holistic assessments are replete with these sorts of aesthetic qualities and judgments that are neither subjective nor objective. Far from being some sort of incomprehensible nuisance, we cannot do without them. Here are some more examples: being grounded, seeing core lift, sensing the balance of spatial masses, seeing lines of order such as horizontals and verticals in the tissues, sensing spirals, waves, vortexes, strains and pulls in the tissues, finding your line (an experience of what the line of gravity is meant to signify), being at odds with your environment, seeing uniform brilliance in the tissues, and so on. These phenomena are excellent examples of aspects of reality that are neither subjective nor objective, but fully there to be perceived by anyone trained to see them.

An important indicator of order to Rolf's way of thinking is her concept of horizontality. She was referring to both the position of the pelvis and also to a perceivable "glow" of horizontality appearing in the tissues. It is less general than beauty, but no less important to our understanding of balance. Its appearance will affect the entire body. In Chapter Nine we will discover why Rolf thought the vertical line of gravity fell short as an indicator of integration and why it needed the addition of orthogonal balance, which includes the horizontal, to capture her vision.

You could expand our understanding of horizontality by coming up with ways to measure horizontality and its effects on structure. You could add to our understanding of the psychobiological assessment type by collating subjective reports about it. To good effect, you could approach most of our fundamental concepts the same way. But the lived experience of horizontality is, as all such concepts are, the prior foundation of any attempt to turn it into an object of scientific investigation. The lived experience of horizontality cannot be reduced to any possible measurement of horizontality, because any particular measurement of horizontality is but a perspective on horizontality, not its lived reality.

From the way Rolf talks about the importance of horizontality, you can see she is interested in more than its measurability; she is also interested in it as a kind of revelation of beauty and wholeness. At the very least, it is both an aesthetic assessment of wholeness and an important aspect of beauty-seeing. She says, "You've got to keep looking, and as you look, you'll suddenly see the horizontal. You've got to keep looking; you've got to evaluate every body that you see. When he gets up and walks does his pelvis look different? And all of a sudden you'll analyze the difference and you'll say, 'Oh my God, yeah, that's Rolf's horizontal.'"[25]

This experience of "all of a sudden" seeing the phenomena is character-istic of the shift of orientation that is required to see in a new way. This shift is an important part of the first step in learning how to see. Recall the giraffe example. On first inspection, it looked like a bunch of ink splotches and squiggles. But when you were instructed to look for a giraffe, suddenly, there it was. Having the concept "giraffe" allowed you to see the squiggles as a giraffe. Although the examples we have been considering are far more complicated and take longer to see, the all-of-a-sudden appearance of the phenomena as something is common to all. When you "get it" the cognitive and the sensory are integrated and you see the phenomena as something— as horizontality or a giraffe, for example.

When all of a sudden the giraffe appeared, it ceased being invisible for you and came into being. It stood out for the first time. You could also say that the squiggles came into meaning. What comes into being (or meaning) is not a pre-given thing just waiting "out there" to be seen. What comes into being is the "appearing-as something." In virtue of appearing-as something (say, a giraffe, horizontality, or an internal or external type), it appears-as meaningful. As we have already seen, com-ing into being is neither subjective nor objective. Led by the power of the thing to manifest itself, we make what was indeterminate determi-nate—we *there* it.

Bringing forth the world is far more complicated than seeing the giraffe. But, in principle, we *there* our world in the same way. Similarly, we also *there* our fundamental assessment concepts, our indicators of order, such as horizontality or finding your line. We learn to see by saturating ourselves for a period of time in all things holistic, by observing a great number of holistic manual therapy sessions, by learning to perceive by means of the assessment types, and by recognizing indicators of order—then, all of a sudden, we integrate concept and sensory experience and finally come to *see*.

What we call seeing in these cases is beyond the ken of the Cartesian onlooker who stands aside and separate from the object of perception. Seeing holistically demands that the seer participate in the very act of seeing, thereby bringing forth wholeness and the beauty of normality. As I suggested above, this kind of lived perception is most akin to aesthetic appreciation: it is about waking up to the beauty of normality.

To the question of how we learn to perceive the beauty of normality, Rolf says, *look and feel*. But this answer is just a way of saying *see it like a Rolfer*, which is just what the beginning student is trying to figure out. The advice she offers is only useful to those who can already see or are on the verge of it: "Rolfers don't need verbal feedback. As you observe more, all kinds of things speak to you.... For me, he [a client] is not something different. When I am Rolfing, he and I form one for at least the time that I'm working. Look and feel. A guy walks in displaying all kinds of things that talk to you. You don't need feedback—you need to look at what's there."[26] Eventually, you will gain an intuitive appreciation of it. Then, you will just *see* it. Not only that, you will also embody it. Notice that learning to see beauty, horizontality, or other similar concepts of order requires a practice of quiet contemplation and the ability to become one with your client. "Yes," says the beginning student, "but how do I make the turn into the kind of seeing that will allow me to take this advice?" Notice that Rolf says that the client and practitioner form one for at least the time of the session. Forming one with the client is an important aspect of what we call "shifting your orientation or intentionality."

If you want to change a dysfunctional structure, Rolf says, "Insist that it get itself into a position which, in your mind's eye, you recognize as the normal. (This is the reason why Rolfers have to sit and listen so much—in order to find what is normal.) When you see it, you can begin bringing the body toward it."[27] You must spend time contemplating the human body as it shows itself to you. To come to know normal you must saturate yourself with the phenomena of holism by quietly observing session after session after session, until finally you *see* order or its lack.

Even though a great many of our assessments are of the aesthetic kind, holistic practitioners also depend upon many different kinds of objective assessment as well. We try to make these assessments without falling into the tendency objective assessments have of viewing the body as a soft machine. Qualitative assessments tend to be about wholeness and relationship. Objective assessments tend to pass over wholeness in favor of finding symptoms and performing measurable assessments. Objective assessments are important to every form of therapy. But because they are often based on conceiving of the body as an assemblage of parts, they tend not to be attuned to interdependent relationships that characterize holistic processes. As a result, at times they miss how the whole responds to both dysfunction and manual therapy. An obvious exception to the problems surrounding holism and its measurement is John Cottingham's elegant holistic research, which uses a vagal tone monitor to measure integration.[28,29,30,31]

The practice of holistic manual therapy demands that "the body as a whole must be balanced. For example, you cannot get movements into a sacrum until you've gotten balance up through the thorax. Realizing this gives you a very different picture of how a totality integrates."[32] The body clearly is not a machine cobbled together from pre-existing parts. The body at one level is a relationship of relationships appropriating the relationship of gravity. Thus, Rolf says, "I'm dealing with problems in the body where there is never just one cause. I'd like you to have more reality on the circular processes that do not act in the body but that are the body. The body process is not linear, it is circular; always, it is circular. One thing goes awry, and its effects go on and on and on and on. A body is a web connecting everything with everything else."[33] The circular wholeness of the body cannot be easily grasped in the narrow confines of objectivity or subjectivity alone. But it can be experienced with an eye that is tuned to the aesthetic.

These comments are all well and good, but unfortunately they only raise the same pressing questions again. How do we experience beauty? How do we wake up to it? How do we become tuned to the aesthetic? How does the advice "look and feel" help us to see? Clearly, beauty is not something that we can measure. Nor is its way of being very obvious. Calling it subjective also misses the mark. What kind of presence is this, that is neither subjective nor objective, yet can feel so intensely *there* when you contemplate it? It is important to understand and appreciate the richness and depth of knowledge and feeling that this kind of lived experience can call forth and know that your experience is not simply a subjective fantasy.

Whether you are talking about the beauty of a flower, a work of art, or a Rolfed body, beauty in every form is a pre-objective, immeasurable presence that presences with the kind of autochthonous, determinate features that invite and enable you to see it. Knowing that it enables you to see it, you must keep looking (quietly contemplating and feeling the situation) until it makes itself known to you, until you see it as something. Rolf's aesthetic assessment of beauty is the result of the same kind of practiced seeing found in phenomenology and Goethe's approach—a dynamic way of perceiving the beauty of normality. Thus, with some justification, we can say that the Rolfer's eye, the phenomenologist's eye, and the artist's eye are the same eye.

The Exercise: There-ing It

At some point, it finally became clear to me that we needed a procedure for training perception. If only we had a step-by-step procedure, we could add it to the saturation method, and we would finally have a way to teach and practice the Rolfer's way of seeing. As it turns out, a little over two centuries ago Goethe discovered just what we have been looking for—a step-by-step procedure for training perception.

Let's begin with the flower and initiate our appropriation of Goethe by first reducing his procedure to its barest bones and filling in the details as we go. Goethe recommends that we engage in what he calls *active seeing* and *exact sensorial imagination* (or, if you prefer, *exact intuitive perception*). In active seeing, we direct our attention to examining the details of the sensuous presence of the flower by means of a sensory/feeling/pre-conceptual openness. Active seeing suspends the verbal/analytic/intellectual mind by directing attention to sensory experience. Then, in exact sensorial imagination, we create a space for the flower in our imagination and lived body by visualizing what we just received/perceived. Next, we check our image with the flower and add and correct what we missed. We do this over and over again, oscillating between active seeing and exact sensorial imagination, until finally the wholeness of the flower appears and lives in us.

We become participants "in the phenomenon instead of onlookers who are separate from it. When we return to the sensory encounter with the phenomenon, we will find that our senses are enhanced and we begin to become aware of the more subtle qualities of the phenomenon. As we follow this practice of living into the phenomenon, we find that it begins to live in us. Whereas the intellectual mind can only bring us into contact with what is finished already, the senses—enhanced by exact sensorial imagination—brings us into contact with what is living, so that we begin to experience the phenomenon dynamically in its coming into being."[34]

It is important to recognize that there is a significant difference between this kind of enhanced seeing and everyday perception. Everyday perception and enhanced perception are both forms of seeing-as. As such, both are saturated with the cognitive. The critical difference is that enhanced perceiving, where the phenomenon lives in us and we in it, must be cultivated by practice. Enhanced seeing is a participatory perception that arises from practicing active seeing and exact sensorial imagination. Everyday perception does not require this kind of conscious cultivation.

If you wish, you can work your way up to people by practicing with plants first. But at this point we will begin by working with people.*

First, find a partner to practice with, preferably a holistic somatic practitioner. To create an exercise we can practice, we need to simplify the process. Think of what we are envisioning as tiny mini-sessions. The idea is to learn this way of seeing on a small scale until you "get it," and it becomes second nature. When it becomes second nature, you can see this way without having to think about each step. As a result, your sessions will naturally go faster. Interestingly, more experienced practitioners are likely to think that they are already doing something very much like what Goethe prescribes. In fact, they probably are. The difference is that Goethe's way is far more explicit than most practitioners' way. The fact that some practitioners sense a similarity only lends further support to the claim that these ways of seeing are the same.

However, before we go any further, we need to underscore an important point that is absolutely crucial for getting good results. This point cannot be stated too strongly or enough: before you do anything else, your very first act must be to shift your orientation or intentionality from an onlooker experiencing the world through abstractions of the analytic/verbal mind to becoming a participant in the lived perception of the

---

*Here is an interesting report from a student who practiced Goethe's method with a plant: "After having spent time observing various Nettles, going to and from them, eventually I was returning to them and feeling like I was meeting an old friend. One day I sat down with a particular Nettle, sat in a patch of many others, I felt a really strong 'star'-like quality. It is very hard to describe but it felt like this enormous spreading, shining sensation—like an expanding force of intense energy. I intuited it as a gesture of the wholeness of the plant. A wholeness that I could then recognize in parts of the plant such as the force of the 'sting' that you feel when touching the small syringe-like 'stinging' hairs; the shape and expression of the thousands of tiny hairs seemingly bursting out of the plant with this immense energy; the pattern spikes on the leaf edges which feel like they are dynamically spreading outward with purpose. The whole plant felt like a star that was shining. A wonderful experience to participate in." This report is from Henri Bortoft, *Taking Appearances Seriously: The Dynamic Way of Seeing in Goethe and European Thought* (Edinburgh: Floris Books, 2012), 175–176.

world. You must shift your orientation to allowing what is to show itself. You simply get out of the way by dropping your self and simultaneously expanding your perceptual field to allow the opening of a loving space. Just allow the spaciousness to appear with no thoughts of trying to change your client for the better. The clarity and safety of this clearing makes it possible for the being of your client to wordlessly reveal his or her troubles to you. This shift is actually a kind of intervention, which, all by itself, can create change. Remember that Rolf recognizes this shift when she says that she becomes one with her client.

As I said, the importance of this shift in orientation from onlooker to participant cannot be over-emphasized. It is part of what we mean by shifting consciousness and includes what Bortoft means by, "There has to be a refocusing of attention from what is conceived to the act of conceiving, while engaged in the act of conceiving that which is conceived."[35]

It is the logically prior precondition for seeing—hence, the key to seeing. In emphasizing it, I am making explicit what is often only implicitly presupposed. It is so important for our purposes that I am adding it to the two-step process I first extracted from Goethe. In our approach, it will be considered the first step in a three-step process and the only step that must remain in effect throughout the entire process of seeing. The three steps are 1) shift your intentionality or orientation from onlooker to participant, 2) engage in active seeing, 3) engage in exact sensorial imagination. Go back and forth between active seeing and exact sensorial imagination until whole phenomena begin to appear and make sure that you remain in the role of a participant throughout.

In the simplest of terms, the exercise looks like this: completely open yourself, body and all, to your colleague, and with the help of your senses (all of them, where appropriate) experience in detail the sensory qualities of your partner and feel the mood that comes with it. As a Goethean researcher says,[36] allow your way of seeing to be shaped by what you're seeing. Close your eyes; visualize what you saw. Re-create in your mind's eye and re-feel in your body the details of the sensory experience of your partner. You might draw what you saw rather than visualize it. You could also imitate how your partner comes to bodily mind-presence with your own body-minding. If you have been visualizing, open your eyes/senses/feeling-nature. If you have been doing something else, come back to the sensory and once more appreciate in detail your colleague's sensuous presence. Close your eyes again. Add any detail to your visualization or your drawing or your whole body gesture that you missed the first time or correct something you may have distorted. Open your eyes/senses/feeling-nature again to the sensuous presence of your partner. Close your eyes and visualize again. Continue engaging in the practice of active seeing and exact sensorial imagination until the wholeness of your partner and/or his or her dysfunctional whole patterns emerge. If you see a thwart to wholeness, don't think you must treat it. Just leave it be. If you decide you want to treat it, in one or two moves only, work to change it—see/feel/work big and holistically.

Practicing oscillating back and forth between active seeing and exact sensorial imagination is designed to activate your imagination while taking you progressively deeper and deeper into an experience of the being of your partner. You begin with shifting your orientation and gathering immediate and direct information by means of your senses—not by means of your intellectual/verbal mind. Pay attention and make conscious your first impressions and the mood that accompanies them. Don't lose your orientation shift by rushing ahead into theorizing, explaining, or categorizing. After engaging in active seeing and exact sensorial imagination for a while, you will begin to notice that your sensory experience and your imagination are intensified.

Whereas active seeing perceives things as separate, when you move into exact sensorial imagination, you are in the realm of relationship creating a space for and participating with the being of your colleague. You are taking the dynamic relational character of the whole being into yourself in order to reveal the formative principle or self-organizing character of the being of your colleague. In time, you begin to sense his or her way of being in the world as a kind of core gestural signature. Depending on the person, the core gesture can be very complicated or very simple. When your friend is so far away that you cannot see his or her face, it is what allows you to recognize your friend in how he or she moves or just stands. This core gestural signature is an expression of your friend's fundamental psychobiological intentionality.

As you contemplate the emergence of this whole-being gesture, who he or she is becomes clearer and more defined. This gestural orientation is your friend's way of being who he or she is. It is manifest not just in his or her comportment, but also in all aspects of his or her being. It is not just an action, but action saturated with meaning. Attending to it allows you to more clearly grasp the principle of your friend's self-organization—how he or she forms him- or herself according to him- or herself. When you grasp it, you do not grasp it through words, but through lived perception. Making drawings, imitating in your own body, putting it to music are all useful ways to sketch the formative gesture of your colleague. As you continue this process, you will begin to perceive your colleague's own most sense of self and fundamental impulse to be.

Your ability to make these kinds of assessments is a complicated form of seeing-as, which in turn depends upon your ability to shift your orientation. Just as the concept of the giraffe allowed you to see the squiggles and splotches as a giraffe, the taxonomies of assessment allow you to transform looking into seeing. The more detailed our categories of assessment become, the more we will be able to see and be prepared to see in our clients. As always happens, the resulting enhanced perception will result in new ways of intervening.

As you continue to allow what is to show itself, the wholeness of your colleague's pattern along with his or her patterns of distortion in relationship to the whole come into clearer focus, and suddenly you see-visualize-feel it coming into being as a unified whole. The unified whole that constitutes your perception is the result of integrating the cognitive with your sensory and feeling-nature. At one and the same time, you are one with your colleague's condition because you feel it and separate from his or her situation because you see it. Simultaneously, you feel your colleague's distortions in yourself and see them in his or her body. Your perception is not a matter of having two different perceptions, one in yourself and one of him or her "over there." Rather, your perception is one integrated, unified whole in which you are both separate and one with your colleague. When you can feel aspects as well as see them, your ability to read your client's emotional and psychobiological orientation is much more accurate than when you deduce them from visual patterns displayed by your client's body. When you perceive your client's structural problems and comportment as sad and angry, you are see-feeling by means of the integration of your cognition, senses, and feeling-nature. Unlike deducing emotions from visual patterns, you are seeing directly what your client is going through.

Now switch places with your colleague and go through the same three-step process with him or her. If this exercise is successful, you will transform your seeing from that of an onlooker to that of a participant. If you continue this participatory practice of seeing, you will probably be amazed by what shows itself to you. Some of what you will see is what you have always seen. But in time you will probably see aspects of the whole person that you did not think were possible.

Conclusion

Just as you cannot find the unity and harmony in a piece of music by breaking it down into individual notes, you cannot find the wholeness of the body when you consider it a thing made of parts. Rolf said, "To a seeing eye, the surface contour of a body delineates the underlying structure. To the practitioner of Structural Integration, the problem becomes one of learning to see spatial masses and to sense their balance."[37] Upon first reading this quotation, you are likely to think, "Well, yeah, every Rolfer knows that." But notice Rolf's entire theory and practice is present with this simple statement. What did she mean by this highly suggestive term, "spatial masses"? Was she just speaking loosely or did she mean something deeper? To wonder about balance is already to wonder about gravity and integration. If there were no such thing as gravity, it would make no sense to ask about balancing spatial masses. Finding balance in gravity is the very core teaching of Rolf. As we consider what is meant by sensing balance and learning to see spatial masses, we are once again drawn into wondering about a qualitative/aesthetic perception. Although she was not adverse to objective assessments (she was a scientist after all), the level of experiential, pre-reflective understanding that Rolf was pointing to cannot be grasped through objective measures alone. To appreciate the lived reality of the knowledge this kind of understanding brings, our indicators of order have to be sensed the way we sense all holistic phenomena, aesthetically.

Before we end this discussion, I want to make a few remarks that require further development. What I call the infusion of the cognitive in perception Goethe and his followers call the work of the imagination. When you are seeing by means of the sensory, you see the separation between things. But when you suddenly see the giraffe or horizontality appear, that is the work of the imagination. The senses reveal the world of separation, while the imagination reveals the holistic world of relationship and connection. We can depict the separate objects given to us through the senses, but we cannot depict the relationships and connectivity of holism. Even though we cannot depict holistic phenomena, we can, through the power of imagination (or cognition), see it. Seeing in the enhanced manner of Rolf or Goethe must be cultivated to where there is an integration of the sensory and the imagination (cognition). When integration is achieved, we experience separation and the relationship and connectivity of holism simultaneously in one simple act of enhanced perception. Through the practice of exact sensorial imagination, the senses are also enhanced. As a result, our enhanced senses make it possible for us to participate in the living presence of the phenomenon and experience it coming into being.

There is more to Goethe's approach than I have sketched here. The complete explication would require a lengthy delineation of his discovery of the ur-phenomenon.*

---

*I have begun this explication in two articles: "Orthotropism and the Unbinding of Morphological Potential," *Rolf Lines* 29, issue 1 (2001): 15–24; "Patterns That Perpetuate Themselves," *Journal of Structural Integration* 37, issue 3 (2009): 23–30.

Where Goethe sees two factors at work in perception—the sensory and imagination—I see a third. I call it our feeling-nature. I encourage you to continue on this path of perception well beyond the integration of the cognitive (imagination) and sensory to the point where you can also integrate your feeling-nature. If you pursue this path of perception long enough, you will discover something truly amazing. When you integrate your feeling-nature with the cognitive (imagination) and the sensory, your perceptual vitality and acuity will be enhanced and your overall skill level (including your perceptual skills, of course) will be suddenly greater and more effective. Not only that, if you keep on keeping on, your feeling-nature will continue to be released from its fixations and conflicts, and you will continue to wake up to your freedom.*

What I have attempted here is a work in progress. It is by no means the final word. I invite you to practice this little exercise to see where it takes you. Keep your boundaries clear, your heart open, your perception immaculate, and practice, practice, practice, practice.

---

*For more on feeling-nature, see my book *Mind Body Zen* (Berkeley: North Atlantic Books, 2010).

CHAPTER 8

Sentient Body

This chapter is about deepening our understanding of holism and how it relates to manual therapy. It is also a critique of certain aspects of metaphysical dualism. The core idea that stands at the heart of metaphysical dualism is the incommensurability thesis. It stipulates that mind and body are mutually exclusive. Since metaphysical dualism arrives at its view of exclusivity by mischaracterizing the nature of both body and mind, the arguments presented here begin by first unraveling the mistaken view that the body is a soft machine.

The first argument is called the "argument from biological organization." It demonstrates that the body is not any kind of machine because the organization of machines and human bodies are radically different from each other. The second argument is called the "argument from corporeal reflexivity." It shows that the ability of living creatures to sense themselves sensing is a capacity forever denied machines. Nature's living reflexive flesh is of an entirely different order than the hardware of machines. This particular difference between flesh and machine not only demonstrates that the body is not any kind of machine, but it also provides good reasons to reject the incommensurability thesis and finally free our perception, thinking, feeling-nature, and senses from the Cartesian hegemony. The third argument of this chapter is called the "argument from evolution." It shows how any organism whose mind and body were mutually exclusive in the way specified by dualism would be an impossible organism. There is another important argument that belongs with the three discussed here. It has already been discussed in Chapter Six. It demonstrates the self-defeating nature of Descartes's metaphysical dualism and how Descartes conflates a causal account of perception with a phenomenological description. The final argument we will consider suggests the mind-body problem, with respect to the possibility of mind and body interacting, is a pseudo-problem.

The underappreciated differences between machines and living bodies support two rather significantly different ways to practice manual therapy. We will take this point up in our discussion of holism. Since the arguments presented here will be strengthened by a discussion of holism, we will look at holism in some detail first.

The Greater Whole Has No Parts to Sum

Unfortunately, holism has become a buzz word that is typically applied thoughtlessly to practices that are not holistic. There are practitioners who think that by massaging the whole body they are engaging in a holistic practice. It is also common these days to find clinics claiming to be holistic that have done nothing more than gather a number of corrective practices under one roof. But, unless there are practitioners who understand holism, no amount of cobbling together second-paradigm practices will ever add up to a holistic clinic. Since the concept of holism is so often misused and abused, we must be clear about what we mean by holism and biological order.

As a way to begin thinking about holism and biological order, consider again an analogy from Merleau-Ponty: "In a soap bubble as in an organism, what happens at each point is determined by what happens at all others. But this is the definition of order."[38] This kind of order is at the heart of and the foundation of any holistic system. Thus, the fundamental principle of holistic intervention is reflected in the soap bubble analogy: "No principle of intervention can be fulfilled unless all are." Because what happens at one point happens at all others, the shape and functioning of the whole body can either limit the effect of our interventions or enhance them. If we introduce changes the body as a whole cannot adapt to, our intervention will fail and we may create difficulties elsewhere. On the other hand, just a few interventions can have profound global effects on the whole structure if they are carefully chosen by a practitioner with an eye for the whole.

Our culture, including our philosophy and science, is under the spell of a machine ontology. But when we break the spell, we discover something surprisingly obvious: *the way your body is organized is nothing like the way even the most complicated machine is organized.* Since the mechanistic ontology understands organic order as mechanical order, it utterly fails to understand the organization of the living body and completely fails to understand the nature of holism. As a result, it supports a way of delivering therapy that is often and necessarily incomplete.*

The corrective practitioner sees the body as an assemblage of localized parts and thus tends to pass over what is essential to the holistic approach: the nexus of interdependent relationships that characterizes living wholes. In organic wholes the relationship of "parts" to the whole is quite different from that of a machine. Consider an analogy to a hologram plate.[39] If you were to break a hologram plate, numerically you would end up with a number of fragments. Remarkably, however, you would discover that each fragment showed the original complete image. Numerically, there are many fragments, but in point of fact there is only one image. In contrast, if you were to break a machine or tear a photograph to pieces, you would be left with broken parts or torn pieces. But nowhere would you find anything comparable to the original whole phenomenon.

In this respect, living wholes are like a hologram plate—the whole comes to presence in each aspect of the whole and each aspect comes to presence in the whole. Furthermore, each aspect is distributed throughout the whole. Thus, with respect to living wholes, there is nothing more fundamental to the order and makeup of the whole than the whole itself.

---

*My criticism of the mechanistic ontology and the kind of therapy it supports should not be taken to mean that I believe a mechanistic approach to biology is altogether wrongheaded. I have no objection to the methodology of trying to understand biological processes through mechanistic models. What I object to is the unsupported idea that all living creatures are nothing more than machines. This latter view is metaphysics, plain and simple, not science. As we saw earlier, it results from confusing methodology with ontology.

As a result, every aspect of the organism exists for and by means of every other aspect, and every aspect enters into the constitution of every other aspect of the organism.

The corrective practitioner is not taught to see with holistic eyes or think holistically. Due to years of training in a mechanistically oriented science, the corrective practitioner is constrained to see the body as a thing made of parts and dysfunction as isolated symptoms. As a result, he or she is somewhat blind to the relational character of dysfunction, or what I call order-thwarters. The mechanistic framework prevents the corrective practitioner from looking for the larger pattern, of which the order-thwarter is but a modification. It also prevents him or her from grasping the chain of dysfunctional dependencies and tendencies to which the order-thwarter is related while simultaneously occluding how the larger pattern is intrinsically connected to the whole body in relation to each person's particular struggle with gravity.

Since the piecemeal way in which the corrective practitioner treats symptoms does not take account of the relational character of living wholes, he or she does not fully appreciate how an intervention in one area of the body can be limited or augmented by what happens in many areas of the body at once. Consequently, corrective practitioners tend to overlook how well or poorly the whole body responds to injury or their interventions. This oversight also undermines their ability to determine the appropriate order in which interventions are delivered.

Lacking the ability to perceive living wholes and how they respond to injury or intervention and seduced by the mechanical ontology, the corrective practitioner does not have a coherent, rational way to answer the three questions of therapy: "what do you do first, what do you do next, and when are you finished?" For example, remember the question the omniscient manual therapist put to the student who worked according to the strategy, "treat the worst first." He asked the student, if a client presents with any number of equally difficult symptoms, how do you decide which one to treat first? Also, the corrective practitioner's client evaluations and treatment plans are often incomplete because they are missing the response of the whole body. The mechanical perspective at the heart of the corrective approach is of no use in trying to decide these issues. Why? Quite simply, the body does not respond to negative forces or positive intervention the way a machine does. Bodies and machines are organized differently.

In contrast to the corrective practitioners, holistic practitioners see the body, mind, and spirit as one unified whole. Their goal is to bring harmony, balance, and morphological integrity to the whole person in relation to the environment. The purpose of therapy is more encompassing than simply getting rid of symptoms. You can easily see this purpose exemplified in the holistic practitioner's desire to enhance the whole person by getting him or her right with gravity. They accomplish this goal by removing in the appropriate order the order-thwarters that diminish our organism's intrinsic ongoing drive to enhance, develop, mature, and become itself (what Metchnikoff, the father of immunology, called orthobiosis). Clients do not get fixed or cured. Rather, they gain a kind of structural maturity in which there is no longer any place for their troubles to reside. Order is not imposed upon clients. It is uncovered.

Symptoms* are seen as order-thwarters. They are treated as a modification of a larger pattern or relationship that is out of balance with the whole. Because order-thwarters, such as back pain, for example, interfere with the goal of achieving integration, they may be addressed both correctively and holistically. But, for the most part, symptoms as order-thwarters are seen as a modification of a larger pattern of relationships.

For example, imagine a kink in a curly telephone cord. Since the kink is a modification of the wire, if you want to get rid of the kink, you have to straighten out the wire, not just fiddle with the kink. In a similar way, symptoms are modifications of a larger pattern that must be addressed if the symptom is to disappear.

---

*The word *symptom* can be understood in at least three ways: 1) "a sign of something else such as a disease state," 2) "fixation (lack of appropriate continuity)," or 3) "somatic dysfunction." I mean *symptom* in the second and third senses, and I use fixation and somatic dysfunction interchangeably. The first sense is used by the medical profession because it deals with disease. Manual therapy is not about disease.

Holistic interventions aim at bringing the order-thwarter back into appropriate relationship with the whole, including the environment. Working with the wholeness of the body and its nexus of relationships is essential to the holistic approach and the foundation for lasting change. Since the goal of holistic work includes bringing the whole body right with gravity, the kinds of techniques required to reposition whole segments of the body are quite different in scope and application when compared to corrective techniques, which are typically limited to local and isolated areas in the body. Remember, as a matter of course, the holistic practitioner can accomplish the goals of the relaxation and corrective approaches, but relaxation and corrective approaches cannot accomplish the goals of the holistic approach, except by accident.

When we look at the actual practice of experienced therapists, we will discover that many of them do not limit themselves to working in one paradigm only. With enough experience many practitioners start seeing holistically. As a result, they work with larger relationships and patterns rather than just isolated symptoms. As their experience deepens, they develop the wisdom to evaluate the global effects of injury and intervention. As a result, they often find themselves naturally working in a holistic way at times, even though their orientation remains that of a corrective practitioner.

Holism and Organic Order

Clearly, living creatures are not assembled from isolated thing-parts. Organisms come into being from living tissue and nothing in their process of coming to be is the least bit comparable to being put together or assembled. Biological order is self-organized and developmental; it is not an order assembled from the outside with pre-shaped parts. We do not say, for example, a baby is being assembled in the womb. We say a baby is developing in the womb. Organisms develop. Machines are assembled and have no intrinsic developmental potential. Mechanical order and developmental order could not be more different.

Strictly speaking, the body does not have parts, at least not in the same sense a machine has parts. Since the body is not made of stand-alone parts, it obviously cannot be considered an assembled structure. Since the body is not made of parts that exist independently from the body, the expression, "The whole is greater than the sum of its parts," is nonsense, at least with respect to living organisms. A more accurate way to make this point would be the greater whole has no parts to sum.

The body is a self-sensing, unified, seamless, developmental, self-organizing whole in which no one aspect or detail is any more fundamental to the makeup and organization of the whole than the whole itself. Unlike a machine, which has no developmental potential, every detail of the organism, whether it is an organ, a bone, or a myofascial structure, is an unmistakably clear, although differently formed, expression of the same self-shaping wholeness and biological identity. Every aspect of an organism is an expression of its self-organizing unified wholeness; every aspect of the organism exists for and by means of every other aspect; and every aspect enters into the constitution of every other aspect of the organism. The whole is expressed in every aspect and every aspect is spread throughout the whole. Each aspect of the body is what is because it stands in relationship not because it stands apart as its own being. You are not an aggregate of pre-shaped parts that lie side by side. Every aspect of your psychobiological nature is a matchless manifestation of your self-shaping, unified, developmental wholeness.

To appreciate the profound difference between mechanical and biological order, consider the ability of the body to communicate with itself at multiple levels. Since the body is a unified, seamless, self-organizing whole in which everything is related to multiple interdependent relationships, communication is one aspect of the body's internal milieu and hence intrinsic to every aspect of the organism. Unlike a machine where communication among parts is made possible by connecting them with other parts, communication among all aspects of a living whole is inherent to the whole.

Rolf said that structure implies relationship. Thus, what we are tempted to call parts are better understood as relationships that are related to many other interdependent relationships. Thus, we can say that the body is actually a relationship in which all relationships are related. The prevailing notion of body parts is an abstraction that does not exist in nature. Organic order is developmental, self-organizing, interconnected, and relational—hence, holistic. To appreciate this interconnected relational whole, imagine the body as a vastly complicated system of mirrors in which each mirror mirrors the others mirroring the whole.

Consequently, holistic somatic therapy must be alert to many interdependent relationships because, as Merleau-Ponty's soap bubble analogy indicates, what happens in one place is determined by what happens in every place. Taking account of interdependent relationships that are characteristic of living wholes requires determining the appropriate order in which various order-thwarters and dysfunctional relationships are to be released in a principled way.

Before we leave the discussion of holism I want to mention one last important point about the relational nature of living wholes. It comes from Mae-Wan Ho's investigations into the interface between biology and quantum mechanics. It succinctly gives voice to the experience of the unified wholeness of the body and how it is capable of intelligently responding as an orchestrated coherent whole to appropriate, but often minimal, interventions. She demonstrates that not only is the body a liquid crystalline continuum organized around a midline, but it is also a form of coherent energy that produces laser-like oscillations. Amazingly, Ho has also found a way to take pictures of the living crystalline continuum.[*,40]

The point she makes is important. She warns us not to think of coherence and wholeness as uniformity where every level is doing the same thing. Rather, she suggests we imagine biological organization as a huge jazz super-orchestra where new parts are continuously and spontaneously

---

*For more information on this fascinating subject see the following two books by James L. Oschman: *Energy Medicine: The Scientific Basis* (Edinburgh: Churchill Livingston, 2000); and *Energy Medicine in Therapeutics and Human Performance* (Philadelphia: Butterworth Heinmann, 2003).

being made up and improvised, where each individual player enjoys complete freedom of expression, but where everybody remains perfectly in step and in tune with the whole. In biological organization the individual players, whether an individual organ, cell, tissue type, or system, have individual frequencies that all combine to create a harmonious collective frequency that is an integrated, unified whole. If these frequencies are disturbed and the body is incapable of entraining them back to normal, then order-thwarters, dysfunction, and disease occur.

Corporeal Reflexivity

Spelling out what is meant by corporeal reflexivity will provide us with two useful results. One is a compelling argument against the mechanomorphic view that the body is a soft machine and the other is a way to show that the incommensurability thesis is false. Let's look at how corporeal reflexivity provides an argument against construing the body as a soft machine first.

It is common in science and evolutionary theory to construe living organisms, including human organisms, as an exquisitely and hierarchically organized but cobbled together collection of little machines. With this unquestioned assumption firmly in place, theorists set about distinguishing the animate from the inanimate. One of the more important distinctions is the incredibly complex hierarchical organization of living organisms, which produces powers not found in inanimate matter, such as self-organization; the capacity to form boundaries; the capacity to respond, to grow, to differentiate, to replicate, to maintain a steady-state balance or homeostasis by means of complex control, communication, and feedback systems; and many more. Researchers in artificial intelligence and artificial life have already modeled some of these characteristics in machines and are increasingly confident that all characteristics of life, including those mentioned above, can either be given a mechanical explanation or be realized in a mechanical form.

But there is one feature of living organisms that is not easily conceptualized as a mechanical phenomenon, and that is the capacity for self-sensing, also known as corporeal reflexivity. All living organisms, even one-celled organisms, have some perceptual ability. With that ability comes the capacity of an organism to sense itself sensing. Clearly, a one-celled organism has no reflective sense of self. But it does have a kind of perceptual sensitivity and, with the creation of its own boundaries, a rudimentary unreflective, anonymous identity that allows it to distinguish itself from what is not itself. Knowing what is me and what is not has practical consequences: in the assimilation of another organism an amoeba must be capable of distinguishing between itself and what it is digesting, otherwise it might digest itself. As Gregory Bateson pointed out,[41] inanimate matter reacts to stimuli, but living beings respond. Kick a rock and you get a rather predictable reaction. But kick a person or a gorilla and you are likely to get a variety of rather disturbing responses.

There are those who might think this ability to respond and distinguish between self and other is not really such a big deal. Consider a thermostat, for example. It is a rudimentary kind of machine that is capable of changing its responses to the environment. And if that is not convincing enough, just consider the existence of those sophisticated, remote sensing robots that are capable of responding to specific environments in rather surprising ways. Given what researchers in artificial life and artificial intelligence have accomplished so far in making "responsive" machines, you might be tempted to conclude that it is only a matter of time before we create responsive machines that begin to emulate more and more of what we easily recognize as consciousness. Because of the advances in these fields, you might even believe, like so many scientists, that every characteristic of life will ultimately yield to a mechanical explanation and a mechanical realization. If we can create a mechanical heart that manifests the functioning of a human heart, then it seems more than reasonable that someday we could create mechanical minds.

These considerations suggest that the word "respond" could be extended to cover how many of our existing machines function. Nevertheless, extending the meaning will not change the fact that the critical difference between how a machine and a living organism respond to or perceive their environment lies in self-sensing. A thermostat does not sense itself sensing. In responding to and perceiving its world a living organism does something that no machine has so far accomplished, or will ever accomplish—it senses itself sensing its environment. Self-sensing is inherent to life. It is a fundamental feature of how all living beings perceive, and this capacity is not found in inanimate matter or among our most sophisticated machines. So far no researcher has thought to mechanically model self-sensing. If it ever occurs to anyone to try, however, they will not succeed. Corporeal reflexivity is not something of which machines are capable. It cannot be programmed and the hardware is all wrong.

Living creatures are not composed of little macros or robots, and mind or consciousness is not "the mere effect of a mindless cascade of mechanical processes," as Daniel Dennett claims in his wonderful philosophical explorations into Darwinian thinking.[42,43] Why? The argument from biological organization and the argument from self-sensing (corporeal reflexivity) show clearly that machines and living organisms are organized quite differently. No form of mechanical ordering of smaller machines will produce a larger self-sensing machine because self-sensing is not a mechanical event. Self-sensing and perception are inseparable activities, which are, in turn, an inseparable feature of the self-organization of living beings.

To topple metaphysical dualism, we have yet to show why mind and body are not mutually exclusive. As compelling as our arguments are, they only cast doubt on one half of metaphysical dualism, the body as soft machine. They are not powerful enough to dissolve the theory once and for all. In particular, we have not solved the problem of how mind and body interact. At best, the arguments only entitle us to say what the body is not. Just knowing that the body is not a machine does not tell us what body and mind are. Unfortunately, we are still laboring under the incommensurability thesis. We still need a way to show that mind and body are not mutually exclusive and thus make sense of their interaction. In order to prepare for a more powerful argument against the mutual exclusivity of mind and body, let's try to first understand and deconstruct the appeal of dualism.

Why Dualism?

We are in possession of two remarkable powers that contribute to the origin of self and to our mistaken belief in a nonphysical form of consciousness separate from our body. They are the ability to use language and the ability to step out of the flow of pre-reflective lived experience and reflect on it. This ability to re-present experience to ourselves linguistically and reflectively is what gives rise to our experience of having a separate self. Since I am able to step back from and reflect on what I just experienced, I can claim this body, all these energies, feelings, sensations, perceptions as my own. I can know and say to myself this is me and recognize that the objects of my perception are not me.

When we try to re-present to ourselves that which knows and perceives the world, we are struck on how that which perceives the world and senses itself sensing cannot be present to itself the same way that the objects of our world can. For example, I perceive the book in front of me, I turn it around it my hands, I smell its newness, I can measure it and weigh it. But when I try to grasp that which senses the book, I cannot do it in the same way. I can certainly turn my attention toward that which perceives the book in the same way I turn my attention to any object of attention. But I cannot hold myself before myself in the way I can hold a simple object before myself.

This self that knows and perceives a world has no shape or outline. I cannot weigh my consciousness or determine its circumference, and I cannot draw a picture of it. Although I do not live my body as a simple object that merely takes up measurable space, I can step out of the flow of pre-reflective experience and treat it that way. I can narrow my experience of my body and treat it like a simple object. I can weigh my body, for example, before going on a diet. Since we can reify our body as an object that takes up measurable space but cannot perceive the perceiver in the same way, we are continually tempted to imagine that consciousness must be a non-bodily, nonphysical thing that has a different ontological status than our body. When we contemplate this feature of our nature and improperly describe it according to Cartesian presuppositions, naturally we are led to embrace a view of mind or consciousness that is defined by excluding anything bodily as well as accept a view of the body that excludes anything having to do with mind.

This mistake is easy to make. We have already brought this view under some scrutiny. We have seen that it is not always appropriate to call something subjective because it is not objective. Consider, for example, what might be called a style of comportment. We recognize each other in the unique ways we walk, gesture, and express ourselves, but these unique styles of comportment cannot be treated as things that take up measurable space. They are as much a part of our perceived world as rocks, apples, and books. Recall our discussion of beauty and aesthetic assessments, for example.

Although we cannot depict, weigh, or find the circumference of beauty or of a style of comportment, it does not follow that they are some sort of mysterious nonphysical something or other that exists in another realm of being. But when it comes to trying to grasp our own consciousness, we are all too ready to accept Descartes's narrowly conceived definitions and conclude that our mind is separate from our body and that mind is some sort of nonphysical ghostlike phenomenon. As it turns out, the discovery of the reflexivity of flesh (corporeal reflexivity) profoundly undercuts this way of thinking by providing a counterexample to the incommensurability thesis. Before we explore the nature of reflexivity and its relevance to our critique of metaphysical dualism, let's take a closer look at how we arrive at the mind-body problem and how the problem is described. How does the mind-body *distinction* become the mind-body *problem?*

How a Distinction Becomes a Problem

Like so many philosophical conundrums, the mind-body problem seems like a trick question. We can state the problem succinctly: if body and mind are mutually exclusive, how do they interact? Something smells fishy already and the more you think about it the more entangled you become. The mind-body *distinction* becomes the mind-body *problem* the minute we embrace the incommensurability thesis, which stipulates in no uncertain terms that mind and body are mutually exclusive. For example, if the body takes up space and the mind doesn't, how is it possible for a non-spatial entity to affect or be affected by a spatial entity? Whatever is mind is not body and whatever is body is not mind. Without the aid of observation or experimentation, we know ahead of time that no interaction between them can ever be possible—because, by definition mind and body are so radically different from one another that interaction is impossible. The difference between mind and body is made too strong and posed in such a way that no solution is possible.

Consider an analogy. A philosopher announces that he has a philosophical problem he wants to discuss. He lays out the problem in the following way. Suppose there are two beings, Ida and Pingala, who can only express their love for each other if they are in close proximity. Unfortunately, the proximity thesis says that it is impossible for them to ever be in close proximity. "Here's the problem," says the philosopher, "Will it ever be possible for them to express their love?" Given the stipulation of the proximity thesis that says they can never be in close proximity and their being in close proximity is a necessity to express their love, we would surely be flummoxed by such a question and could only reasonably answer, "No, of course not, you have defined the problem in such a way that they can never express their love." To wonder whether they can express their love when close proximity is forever impossible but absolutely necessary is nothing short of bizarre. It is hardly the statement of a philosophical problem that needs a solution.

The setup for the mind-body problem follows the same bizarre path. From the very beginning it is stipulated that mind and body are mutually exclusive. Because they are defined so radically different from each other, the question of their interaction is impossible. After accepting the stipulations, if someone now wonders whether it is possible for the mind and body to interact, the only reasonable answer is, "No, of course not." As long as you accept the incommensurability thesis, mind and body will never be able to interact. They can't. Built into the statement of the problem is the impossibility of interaction. With respect to the problem of interaction, the mind-body problem is manufactured. Like our analogy, it is not a problem that needs solving.

Clearly, the problem lies with the incommensurability thesis. Why do we so readily accept without question the characterization of mind and body as mutually exclusive? It should be clear that once we accept how the incommensurability thesis defines and characterizes mind and body, we will be mired in trying to solve a problem that cannot be solved. Purely as a result of how the problem is defined, no solution is possible and no interaction between mind and body is possible. Are we bamboozled by the incommensurability thesis because the way the distinction is drawn is the only way we can imagine it? If so, the discovery of corporeal reflexivity will show us how to draw the distinction between body and mind without making them mutually exclusive.

Why I Am Not an Object

As long as the assertion that mind and body are mutually exclusive stands uncontested, we will remain saddled with the mind-body problem. Let's back up one more time and describe the appeal of dualism from a different angle. All the difficulties that accompany our attempt to understand our embodiment begin with a simple way of thinking about the body—so simple, in fact, that it seems to be nothing more than unassailable common sense. The assumption is that the body is a mere object.

When I turn my attention to myself, I don't think of myself as a mere object. After all, I am aware. I think. I feel. I dream. I appropriate gravity. Mere objects do not do anything similar. They are not self-movers. They just sit there taking up space. Since I am nothing like that, what I am must be entirely different. Since the essence of who and what I am is not an object, I am not my body. If what I am cannot be measured and it does not take up space, it must have some other kind of ghostlike existence. That ghostlike phenomenon we call mind or soul. Notice how metaphysical dualism naturally and quickly arises with assuming the body is an object.

Biting at the heels of this assumption are all the logical and phenomeno-logical problems associated with the incommensurability thesis.

The key to breaking the spell of metaphysical dualism lies in the rec-ognition that the very first step we took in thinking about our body was actually a critical misstep that sent us careening off in the wrong direc-tion. The body is not what common sense says it is. It is not an object. But what is the body if not an object? The short answer is that the body is sentient. The claim that the body is sentient means that consciousness is rooted in the material reflexive flesh of the body. What we call mind or consciousness in ourselves is an evolutionary elaboration of the capacity for self-sensing (or sentience) that is inherent to all life.

Unfortunately, a clear consensus about the meaning of the word "sen-tience" does not seem to exist. The meanings that hover around it are consciousness, awareness, perception, intelligence, sensation, sensitiv-ity to stimuli, and so on. In considering all these meanings I think it is safe to say sentience means "self-sensing." Even though the sort of self-awareness that we call consciousness in ourselves is astonishing in com-parison to the self-sensing that constitutes the awareness of other forms of life, self-sensing is, nevertheless, the ground from which human con-sciousness evolved. To say that self-sensing is what human consciousness evolved from means that awareness and consciousness began as reflexive flesh. Since reflexive flesh is part of the material world and consciousness arose from it, consciousness does not exist as an immaterial, nonphysical, non-spatial entity. With the insight that consciousness is rooted in the reflexivity of flesh a second insight comes tumbling after—consciousness is part of the material world and mind is a somatic event.

Although they are not separate from each other, we can distinguish *the flesh of self-sensing* from the *act of self-sensing*. The act of self-sensing cannot be measured and cannot be easily located. Since the act of self-sensing is not separate from the flesh of self-sensing, self-sensing takes place in the reflexive material flesh of the body. Hence, sentience is inherent to the material body and is, of course, part of the material world. The act of self-sensing takes place in the material flesh of living organisms. It is an act of the living material body. Under the weight of these considerations, the incommensurability thesis crumbles. Thus, with respect to the interaction between mind and body, there is no mind-body problem. There is only a mind-body distinction.

To simplify and clarify this important argument, let's consolidate our insights into a simple argument form.

1. The body is not an object.
2. The body is sentient or reflexive (i.e., capable of sensing itself sensing).
3. Sentience is the act of the body sensing itself sensing.
4. Sensing oneself sensing is a form of consciousness.
5. Consciousness is a somatic event.
6. Therefore, the incommensurability thesis is false.

If mind is a somatic event, the interaction of mind and body is possible. Both body and mind are two aspects of the same interdependent activity. The idea that body and mind are mutually exclusive must be replaced with the view that they mutually implicate each other.

Starting Over

Since the sentient body has qualities we thought were exclusive to mind, we need to completely rethink the distinction between mind and body. As Buddha said, "The foot feels the foot when it feels the ground." The import of this insight is crucial. It topples the hegemony of metaphysical dualism and the incommensurability thesis. It means that what we call mind exists as a material somatic reflexive event. Flesh and consciousness are two aspects of the same reality. Since they are two aspects of the same reality, their interaction is no longer a problem. With respect to the question of their interaction, the mind-body problem simply evaporates.

As a result of these considerations we must go back to the beginning and rethink the mind-body distinction. The shackles have been thrown off and the incommensurability thesis has been cast aside. Nevertheless, we must be careful not to slip back into the language and blinders of dualism. We will have to get used to the idea that what we used to refer to as mind and body has changed. Now when we say body, we do not mean something that excludes mind; we mean sentient body, a body that has qualities we used to think were inherent only to mind. When we say mind, we are now talking about something that has qualities we used to think were exclusive to the body.

Recall that Merleau-Ponty said that thought is the result of the development of the body's ability to perceive. He was the first to argue that the body is not a mere object. If you accept the view that the body is sentient, then you must also accept that consciousness begins with reflexive flesh. Both propositions deal a deathblow to the incommensurability thesis by showing that mind and body are not mutually exclusive. As a result, we must now be prepared to rethink and clarify the meaning of many of our fundamental concepts. What phenomenology discovered as intentionality, for example, is not a property of some kind of non-bodily transcendental mind, but is very much rooted in the lived-body and its being-oriented-toward-and-being-solicited-by-a-world.

I can make a functional distinction between my body and my world-view, but how I live my worldview is not separate from how I live my body. Mind and body no longer mean quite the same thing. But our new ways of thinking about them are more in keeping with what we regularly notice as manual therapists. Flesh and thought are modifications of the sentient body, not two ontologically separate realities. If we dwell on our own situation, even in the most cursory manner, it is hard to miss how much the suffering of our sentient body actually involves a complex deliquescent intermingling of somatic dysfunctions with conflicted cognitive or psychological processes. These insights require that we begin at the beginning and start all over again.

Starting over begins with no longer being under the spell of the incommensurability thesis. Instead we recognize "mind and body" as two different interdependent expressions of sentience. The sentient body and its environment mutually implicate each other and function together as interdependent activities. Our way of knowing and being in the world is enabled by our environment. At the very least, we must begin with the willingness to expand and relax the traditional limitations of the subject/object distinction. Knowing that what shows itself is sometimes neither subjective nor objective can help keep us attentive and open to what shows itself. Since so many holistic assessments are aesthetic in character, neither subjective nor objective, we especially need to release them from the forceps of a misplaced skepticism and freely explore the kind of seeing from which they emerge. One of the best ways to explore this kind of seeing is to practice the three-step exercise.

Argument from Evolution

Freeing ourselves from the influence of metaphysical dualism is no easy task. When added together, the accumulative effect of our arguments against dualism go a long way toward freeing us from the Cartesian hegemony. They are sufficient to initiate the process of casting the Cartesian worldview aside, making it possible for us to open our eyes to the true beauty that is our home. The last argument we will level against metaphysical dualism is "the argument from evolution." It goes as follows.

By means of natural selection, the sentient body and environment evolve together—not as separate and distinct projects, but as an interdependent unity. Because they are different manifestations of the same evolutionary activity, we see ourselves in our environment and the environment finds itself in us. The evolution of the sentient body and its environment clearly presupposes a working interdependent relationship between mind, body, and the external world. Sentient body, environment, and world all mutually implicate each other and are intertwined expressions of the same evolutionary activity. Since organisms and their environments evolve together, it is not surprising that we find ourselves in a mostly humanely habitable environment in which mind and body function harmoniously.

We are able to be at home and at ease in a world that makes sense to us. Although there is no designer of our world, save natural selection, our world appears designed with us in mind. It is designed with the means to make our world ultimately habitable. When you add to this insight the theory from evolutionary biology that the organism and its environment evolve together, it is reasonable to think that a favorable, enabling environment that supports and enables our way of being is probably the most likely evolutionary outcome.

No humanly habitable world would be possible if the incommensurability thesis were true. Given that organism and environment are interdependently related, and the world enables us to know and be at ease with it, imagining a world saddled with the Cartesian vision of a human being would be next to impossible. The chances of survival for such a severely dysfunctional and ontologically bifurcated creature whose mind and body are so different from one another that neither can interact nor communicate with the other would be slim to none. Evolving a habitable environment for the Cartesian human would be the waste of an environment, even if it were possible. A human being like the one envisioned in the Cartesian worldview is too disabled to find itself at home in any actual environment. Descartes's incommensurability thesis is so powerful that it makes our life and world as we know and live it impossible. Therefore, it can be cast aside.

Conclusion

An interesting way to end this phase of our study of manual therapy is to pose a question for future investigations: can there be a biology of consciousness, does consciousness have a biological basis, or is consciousness forever beyond the reach of science?

This chapter is the culmination of a variety of criticisms, which when taken together add up to the first step in dismantling dualism. There are still a cluster of issues associated with the mind-body problem that I have not addressed, such as the possibility of artificial intelligence, artificial life, and perhaps the most important of all, the very nature of consciousness itself. The question about the nature of consciousness has come to be known as the "hard problem of consciousness."[44] The hard problem is trying to account for subjective experience. We have already run into this difficulty in Chapter Six where it was pointed out that science cannot measure the experience of purple, the taste of strawberries, or the experience of beauty, for example. A neurological account of what it is like to have consciousness is about as illuminating as a chemical analysis of the experience of beauty.

Consider yet another example. Imagine someone who only sees in black and white waking up one day suddenly seeing the world in color. Looking around in amazement, he says, "So that's what it looks like." What is he seeing?[45] It seems no matter how hard we try, science will never be able to account for or capture what it is like to experience color or consciousness. In other words, you cannot reduce a first-person account (I have a pain in my back) to a third-person account (the neurological account of pain by an external observer). Therefore, the hard problem of consciousness is not just a difficult problem we may someday solve. It is profoundly difficult because consciousness and subjective experience can never be grasped by science.

Those philosophers who think that the hard problem will never be overcome are more than likely still under the influence of the incommensurability thesis. As a result, they are still confounded by the notion that mind and body are mutually exclusive and the attendant view that consciousness is some sort of nonphysical ghostlike phenomenon. But since the incommensurability thesis has been shown to be false, it is safe to assume that certain aspects of consciousness are bodily in nature. The fact that we can show that consciousness has a biological basis in reflexive flesh means, at the very least, that *some* (perhaps not all) aspects of consciousness are open to scientific investigation and that a biology of consciousness is a real possibility. In any case, the insight into the reflexivity of living tissue demands a fresh approach to the issue of consciousness.

With these points established, we can finally put the incommensurability thesis and the puzzle of how mind and body could interact behind us and begin looking at the mind-body relationship, consciousness, and our embodiment with new eyes—eyes that have learned to see the body as consciousness. The mystery of consciousness is the mystery of the sentient body.

CHAPTER 9

Appropriating Gravity

Hopefully, we have sufficiently clarified the nature of holism and have shown why the body is not a soft machine to now turn to a discussion of gravity. We have explored the relational organization of living wholes. But we have not yet explored the connection between balance, integration, and gravity. The question of gravity brings us face-to-face with the vital significance of verticality to human life, integration, and holism. Unlike a stack of blocks, which is acted upon passively by gravity, our upright vertical posture appropriates gravity. To say that we appropriate gravity is to say that our upright structure can take advantage of gravity by both organizing itself in gravity and organizing itself to meet gravity. The more balanced our body becomes, the more gravity reinforces our balance. We feel more at home in our bodies and the world and more alive to the solicitations of the world. Rolf said that when the body is integrated in gravity, gravity supports and flows through the body.

You may remember I said that the holistic practitioner attempts to transform the sky not push the stars. As far as metaphors go, this one is not too bad. What is missing is an explicit recognition of the importance of gravity to our understanding of holism.

Let's hear what Rolf has to say about gravity and working with the human body. "To a seeing eye, the surface contour of a body delineates the underlying structure. To the practitioner of structural integration the problem becomes one of learning to see spatial masses and to sense their balance."[46] The core of Rolf's teaching is found in this simple statement about finding balance in gravity. If there were no such thing as gravity, it would make little sense to talk about balancing spatial masses. Merely contemplating what is meant by sensing balance and learning to see spatial masses is enough to suggest that the implications of this simple statement are far from simple. One very important implication concerns the connection between gravity and holism.

If we pursue this connection far enough, we will discover that any definition of holism that leaves out gravity or the environment is incomplete. This oversight adversely affects how therapy is conceived and delivered. To the extent we do not recognize the importance of getting the body right with gravity, we run the risk of compromising the results of our therapy. For example, if a practitioner gets wonderful results with the client's neck and shoulders, but there is not enough support and adaptability for the changes achieved, it is almost certain that the good results will not last.

Lines of Organization

In an effort to grasp this complicated relation to gravity we will begin with some of the more common attempts to articulate the significance of the verticality of the human body, beginning with the line of gravity. Then we will look at what it means to say that the body organizes itself to meet gravity.

A common way to evaluate body alignment and stability is to compare body alignment with the line of gravity. If your line is straight, your organization is good and gravity reinforces your balance. To the extent you deviate from this line, gravity is at war with your body and doesn't flow through as it should. Rolf said it this way, "For a strain free system ..., there must be a vertical alignment of each block's gravitational center; there must also be no rotation or tipping of segments."*,47 Evaluating vertical alignment and stability according to the line of gravity seems simple and straightforward. But it is only simple and straightforward when you are dealing with a stack of blocks where every block is equally dense throughout. When we consider the human body, things are messier. As Advanced

---

*See also Florence P. Kendall et al., *Muscles: Testing and Function*, 3rd ed. (Baltimore: Williams and Wilkins, 1983), 19.

Rolfing Instructor Peter Schwind astutely pointed out, the human body is not equally dense throughout. As a result, it is not possible to establish alignment with a plumb line. Or alternatively, if it were possible to line up the body's weight centers, you would end up creating a rather ungainly, graceless, and oddly shaped body. Just think of how the weight centers might line up in a person with a large potbelly or a very pregnant woman.

Rolf also clearly recognized that the plumb line could not account for certain features of a well-organized body, but not for the same reason as Schwind. She said that the line of gravity with its image of neatly stacked blocks was "an unfinished metaphor" for determining stability and alignment. To those practitioners who primarily evaluate structure by means of the line of gravity, what Rolf says next may be perplexing. "In human bodies, symmetry along all three major axes is the only ultimate answer, not merely alignment in a vertical dimension." She observed that "the human body, when schematized to a set of blocks, shows wider, heavier, bulkier blocks at the shoulder level than near the ground. Our simpler system of blocks did not take our problem [top heaviness] into account."[48] Thus, integration in gravity requires more than the line of gravity. It also includes a lived palintonic symmetry (across the transverse, the coronal, and the sagittal axes). By itself, the line of gravity cannot do the job of providing a norm for balance, stability, and alignment. It also follows that the famous little boy Rolfing logo is not a standard or norm for judging how well integrated a person is. The logo is a representation of a metaphor, not a standard.

In rejecting line of gravity as an indicator for integration in gravity, I am not suggesting that the concept of a line has no place in our evaluation of alignment. Thus, for example, Mae-Wan Ho seems to explicate a concept of a midline that converges with the osteopath's concept of a midline. Recall that Ho discovered that the body is a liquid crystalline continuum and a form of coherent energy. Like all crystals, solid or liquid, it is organized around a central vertical midline that has very little to do with the line of gravity. It develops in us from the first cell division and lays down the path for the development of the notochord and spine, for example. This midline is the fundamental organizing principle of the body discovered by William Sutherland, DO, and cultivated in many forms of Eastern meditation.* The line of gravity is an abstraction imposed on the body from the outside whereas the midline is a dimension of the body itself. What many call the core of the body may well be this primordial midline.

Gravity also brings us face-to-face with the significance of verticality to being upright. Human beings are not just passively affected by gravity. Unlike a machine our upright vertical posture appropriates gravity. Rolf also used another metaphor for a strain-free stable body. She compared the body to tensile structures like a tent or a suspension bridge. She pointed out that it is not the poles that maintain the tent in gravity but the way the fabric and the guy-wires are appropriately stretched across the poles that is responsible for the tent's integrity. In other words, she is again pointing out that integration is a matter of appropriate palintonicity.** In this respect, she said that the body was more like a tent or suspension bridge than a stack of blocks. The tent analogy breaks down, however. While we can agree that the architectural integrity of the body is a function of how the myofascia is appropriately stretched across the skeletal system, it is not the whole story. When we lose consciousness, our bodies do not remain upright. They simply crumple to the ground.

---

*For a fascinating discussion of the nature of midlines and their organizing function see especially the second volume of Franklyn Sills' two-volume work, *Craniosacral Biodynamics* (Berkeley: North Atlantic Books, 2001 and 2004). For the sake of clarity I should point out that even though Mae-Wan Ho does not mention Sutherland's discovery, she clearly articulates the organizing function of the midline. She says, for example, "some global orienting field is indeed responsible for polarizing liquid crystalline phase alignment, and hence, in determining the major body axis"—*The Rainbow and the Worm: The Physics of Organisms*, 2nd ed. (Hackensack: World Scientific Publishing Co., 1998), 166. An example of a structure whose center acts as an organizing axis or core is the well-known donut-shaped torus.

**Rolf was attracted to the German word *Spannung* because it captured many of the experiential and objective meanings with which she was most concerned. *Spannung* can mean span like that of a tensile structure, the relaxed but vital sense of energy we experience during intense moments of creative or meditative activities, the integrative experience of body-mind harmony, etc. Palintonos includes the meanings of *Spannung* and *Zugspannung* but is even broader in its implications. Palintonic harmony also describes the unity of opposition that constitutes the harmony of the wholeness of being and our relationship therein. It is not just a description of how the body is acted upon by gravity and the environment, but more importantly a description of how the body responds to and appropriates gravity and its environment.

The line of gravity may be a useful metaphor with which to begin understanding how our bodies relate to gravity, but in the end it is also misleading. Rather than trying to make a body conform to an external standard such as the line of gravity, a more appropriate way to work is to uncover and cultivate the body's own morphological imperative. Encouraging the verticality that already wants to happen allows the body to find its own way home. The primordial midline function is closer to the true line of integration because it is an intimate and perceivable part of the very organization of the body itself. Unlike the line of gravity, which has no intrinsic perceivable organizing referent in the body and functions like an external abstract standard to which the body is supposed to conform, the midline is inherent to the body and, as a result, a reality practitioners can get their hands on.*

Orthotropism

Rolf said that the body is something built around the line. As long as we do not mean by "line" the line of gravity, this statement can be understood as a metaphor of integration in gravity. But in truth, every inch of the body is striving to unbind its morphological potential by cultivating the vertical. Seeking the vertical is a dance not limited to the midline, or any particular structure, aspect, or organ—it is an activity of the body as a whole.

Although the human form evolved from the animal form and shares the same anatomical structures in common with all mammals, human morphology is quite different. By vertically appropriating gravity human morphology transforms these common animal structures and organizes

---

*For an elaboration of these points and their relationship to the practice of holistic therapy see my following four articles: "Moving toward Our Evolutionary Potential," *Rolf Lines* XXIV, no. 2 (May 1996): 5–23; "Radical Somatics and Philosophical Counseling," *Rolf Lines* XXVII, no. 2 (Spring 1999), 29–40; "Perception and the Cognitive Theory of Life: Or How Did Matter Become Conscious of Itself?" *Rolf Lines* XXVII, no. 4 (Fall 1999): 5–13; and "Orthotropism and the Unbinding of Morphological Potential," *Rolf Lines* XXIX, no. 1 (Winter 2001): 15–23. Also relevant is my book, *Spacious Body: Explorations in Somatic Ontology* (Berkeley: North Atlantic Books, 1995).

them into an upright, self-directed, self-sensing, self-conscious whole that is always striving for verticality. Verticality and consciousness evolved together and are inseparable in the human form. Verticality and consciousness have indelibly shaped our form. From inside to outside, from head to toe, our morphology is forged by our verticality and consciousness.

Consider a few examples. Seen posteriorly, an infant's calcaneus is quite rounded. But with the attainment of a more mature upright form the calcaneus expresses the body's verticality by elongating. Or look at how the human femur contributes to our erect morphology by being more developed and elongated than the femurs of other mammals. Or contemplate the differences between the animal and human cranium. In the human cranium the snout retreats into a face, the jaw ceases to hang heavy as it does in the gorilla, and the upward-striving forces create a cranial vault that is more or less rounded into a peak.

Just think of the myriad self-maintaining, self-shaping activities of the human body and you will see that there must be more to integration than treating the body as a mere thing to be lined up in gravity. Our morphology is shaping and being shaped by a throng of internal and external forces. There are motile forces always at work in the body, the abdominal and thoracic cavities express different pressures, the hollow organs are continually maintaining their shape by means of pushing-out forces, there are emotional ups and downs, there is the continual flow of peptides that agitate and mollify, there are the rhythms of the heart and lungs to contend with, and the shaping of our body by the emotions we have repressed—and all the while our organismic identity and consciousness maintain themselves and their uprightness amidst all these and other forces as well as against a host of perturbations coming from the outside.

This self-defining, self-maintaining, self-sensing capacity of our psycho-biological nature has one feature unique to our upright form, which is fundamental and central to the practice of third-paradigm therapy—the human body's ongoing activity of seeking the vertical. This activity of seeking the vertical can best be captured by the word "orthotropism." "Orthotropism" is composed of "ortho," which means "right," "straight," "upright," "correct," or "vertical," and "tropism," which refers to the tendency of an organism to grow toward or away from something. Thus, as a plant is heliotropic because it grows toward the light, the human body is orthotropic because it grows toward the vertical. But it is important to emphasize that the human body does not just grow toward the vertical; it *seeks* it in every moment. The way the human body is constantly negotiating its verticality is a central activity of its self-organization and self-shaping. The human body is not passively acted upon by gravity; it is constantly appropriating gravity orthotropically. Since verticality is an activity intrinsic to how our morphology lives to express itself, our way of working cannot be a process of imposing verticality and order on the body, but the attempt to activate the body's own orthotropic response. Verticality is not imposed on the body; it is uncovered.

When a body experiences thwarts to its morphological potential, it tries to negotiate its verticality the best way it can. Striving for verticality, it finds a way to get around the order-thwarters by seeking the best vertical compromise it can manage. A good analogy for this compromise is the way a stream flows around a boulder.

By dealing with these order-thwarters in an orderly and systematic manner, holistic manual therapy unbinds the morphological potential in the body so that it can renegotiate its verticality by better organizing itself around its midline. Once we break free of somatic idealism and formulism, our practice is no longer a matter of imposing a template on every person. The holistic, principle-centered decision-making process recognizes that there is no one way that every body expresses its orthotropism. As a result, non-formulistic therapy becomes a holistic attempt to activate the orthotropic effect by finding the best and most systematic way to release the order-thwarters in order to unbind the unique morphological potential that is always living to express itself.

Appropriating Gravity

As we discovered in Chapter Eight, the problem with most attempts to articulate the relationship between our bodies and the Earth is that they assume that the body is a mere thing. The tent and stack of blocks analogies are clearly problematic because they assume the body is a mere thing. Therefore, when we speak of the body's verticality, we are not simply referring to the body as an object but to the orthotropic activity of the sentient body.

To understand, to see, and to feel the reality of what is being discussed here, it would be useful to review the discussion of seeing in Chapter Six and practice the exercise for seeing in Chapter Seven. As practitioners, we want to cultivate order and the vertical as if we were midwives, not as if we were traffic cops.

Not only can you see how orthotropism is expressed in every detail of the form of the human body, you can feel it assert itself when you are working with people. Feeling for the orthotropic effect makes our work easier and gentler. Instead of imposing our will on the body, we wait for the body's response to our touch. We must learn how to feel our way into the person and wait for what the body wants to show us. When the body is recognized, it begins to unravel from its misery. When it finishes unraveling, the tissues soften. But if you wait just a little bit longer, realizing that you are not finished when tissues soften, you notice a wondrous thing—you feel the effect of your touch spreading above and below where your hands are as the body begins to organize itself around the vertical (actually, it also organizes itself around the coronal and transverse planes). When you feel and see this striving for order and verticality coming from within the body itself, you are feeling the orthotropic effect.

Like all living creatures, we are always involved in this self-maintaining activity, constantly defining ourselves in opposition to what is not me. In order for an organism to have a world, it must be capable of meeting what comes its way with a constancy that matches what comes its way. It must continually define itself by maintaining its boundaries. This self-defining, self-making activity is the biological root of psychological boundaries. But unlike other mammals, part of our self-defining activity consists in seeking the vertical. By releasing a restriction in one place, you activate the body's own aspiration to negotiate its verticality anew. Where it fails to negotiate verticality, you see loss of continuity. This dance of verticality is part of what it means to say that the body is not merely acted upon by gravity, but always responding to it. The human body is ceaselessly seeking the vertical in gravity. If we evaluate clients only according to how well they approximate the line of gravity, we will systematically miss how our clients struggle with gravity and finding verticality—and it is immensely important that we don't miss this struggle. Our work will be more effective if we learn how to cultivate the orthotropic effect while we are releasing order-thwarters.

If enough bound morphological potential is unleashed, the body as a whole shifts palintonically. Grounded, it settles down to the Earth and lifts skyward. Seeking the vertical is also about finding the between of the Earth and the sky and balance between the inside (core of the sentient body) and outside. Being grounded and feeling lift is not some vague, ill-defined metaphor. Being uplifted and grounded is a wonderful expression and experience of our body's orthotropic nature. It is also a condition of fluid-flowing, unencumbered, coordinated movement. But experiencing it fully requires disabusing ourselves of the Cartesian worldview.

Using support as an example, let's look more carefully at how the body organizes itself to meet gravity and the environment. If we assess our clients with the eyes of a mechanic, with only the block model, tent analogy, and line of gravity in mind, we will be concerned only with the question of how well their legs are under them. I am not denying the importance of getting the legs under a body. But I am saying that many of our traditional ways of evaluating structure presuppose a mechanistic orientation that occludes something about support just as important as the idea of getting the legs under the body. I am also saying that even if we get the legs under the body, we may not get this deeper kind of connection to the Earth. If we don't get this deeper connection to the Earth, all of our attempts at integration will be limited accordingly.

In your assessment, ask yourself about how your client appropriates gravity. In what way does his or her body organize itself to meet the floor? Is there a soft, responsive, expansive way the body meets and surrenders its weight through the legs to the Earth or are the lower legs stiff and wooden? Problems in support are not just about whether the legs are properly under the body, but also about whether the legs meet the floor in this fluid, responsive, soft way. Like a big soft paw, the feet should easily engage the floor. In the weight-bearing phase of walking the medial arch should flatten a bit, and during the push-off phase it should spring back to its unloaded form, thereby creating a springing effect up through the leg as if the foot subtly bounced off the floor. Imagine the tibia and fibula like a bow with the interosseous membrane stretched between. When the leg meets the Earth, do the bones easily bow apart, thereby absorbing the shock, or does the lower leg respond like one stiff thing?

Now expand this way of looking just a bit more and ask about where your client's orthotropic response is being compromised. How is his or her body organized to meet the Earth? How does your client find the Earth and surrender weight to it? How and where in his or her body does your client fail to find the Earth? Where is the flow of coordinated movement hindered? How does your client move into repose or stress? Does the body sink into the Earth too much or does he or she push away from it? How well or poorly does the body appropriate gravity? Think even bigger than how your client meets the Earth and ask where the body loses its open, expansive response to the world. Does the form seem unable to meet the world and environment or does he or she push too strongly into the world? Where does your client do this in his or her body? Where is your client pulled? Where does your client push? Where is his or her form struggling to express itself? How is movement affected by defensive pushing away or pulling back? How does your client maintain the form that is living to express itself? How your client does this is who he or she is. Look for where and how your client's morphological potential is being bound, about where the morphology that is living to express itself is being thwarted.

How can we become who we are if our morphological potential is thwarted? As I have said many times, freedom is the creative appropriation of limitation, and Rolfing is the creative appropriation of gravity. Our assessments should include looking at the shape of these inherent responses and forms of intentionality, about how the being of the whole person shows up in meeting or failing to meet gravity, the environment, and the world. Don't get lost in a world of joint restrictions and tight myofascia. Give up the detached onlooker orientation and become a participatory percipient. Pretend you are looking at one unified protoplasmic body that can shift its form and density whenever it's required, whether deep or superficial, and you will begin to see these whole somatopsychic body patterns emerging. Show the sentient body how to unbind itself orthotropically and it will reward you with the beauty of flowing, coordinated movement.

Conclusion

Thus, we recognize within the meaning of support there are two ways we can relate to the Earth. One has to do with how well the legs are under the body and the other has to do with how the body is organized to meet the Earth. Not limiting our discussion to support, we can ask the same sort of questions about other dimensions of the body. How well is the thorax under the head, or how do the upward and downward forces meet or deflect one another? How freely does the body appropriate gravity?

If we organize our way of touching the body around activating the orthotropic effect, then the body will release itself the way it needs to and find the best possible structural change for itself. Instead of willfully imposing a template of the ideal body on our clients, we will find ourselves involved in a process of discovery, where we unbind the morphological potential in the way that most suits the individual person we are working with. If you work this way, in conjunction with the principles of intervention, you will see this open, expansive, self-shaping response to the world coming from the body itself. As a result, you will see the shape change that matches what works for the uniqueness of the person's morphology, instead of one that has been imposed on his or her body.

When we touch the body, we do not want to treat it like a thing or object that merely takes up measurable space. The body is not a mere object.

The body is sentient. We want to touch in such a way that the body meets and shows us its patterns of distress. If we drop our self sufficiently enough, when we put our hands on, we become like an innocent child to whom the sentient body willingly reveals itself. Now here is the amazing thing: when we recognize the sentient body in this participatory, pre-reflective way, when we innocently allow it to be what it is, it will seek the order that serves its own unique morphology by itself—we don't initiate the change, the body does. Our first job is to recognize the sentient body in this participatory, pre-reflective way so that the body can initiate how to unbind itself. By working this way, we are tapping into the self-organizing, self-making, reflexive, self-shaping orthotropic nature of our client. When immaculately perceived, the whole person, without thought or will, simply moves toward the next highest level of integration and order it can manage. All we have to do is pre-reflectively allow the sentient body to find its way into activating that orthotropic activity.

CHAPTER 10

In Praise of Subjectivity

This chapter is concerned with finding our way around some of the common stumbling blocks to practicing holistically. Neither Rolf's holistic way of seeing nor aesthetic appreciation can be grasped within the narrowly conceived confines of objectivity (the measurable) or subjectivity (what is only true for me). But if *seeing* holistically is the important skill we think it is, we must learn to embrace it as a legitimate way of perceiving—and practice it. Learning to see as a seasoned holistic manual therapist sees is also about learning to be free.

This chapter also contains a brief sketch of what a refurbished mind-body relationship might look like in the hands of a holistic practitioner. Interestingly, the discussion of biological order inevitably leads to the surprising insight that every imaginable form of medicine or therapy is, at bottom, holistic. Since biological order is holistic, it only stands to reason that the appropriate treatment of our ills must also be holistic. Equally surprising is how the majority of manual therapists continue to practice their art in the second paradigm, altogether ignoring or misunderstanding holism.

The Felt-Experience of Concepts

There are many ways to become a better holistic manual therapist. But one that is probably never mentioned, even though it is foundational, is getting free of the hegemony of the Cartesian worldview. Because the Cartesian way of thinking has such a hold on us at many levels, getting free of it is not easy. We must bring clarity to not only our dysfunctional, sedimented ways of thinking, but also to how we have shaped ourselves to see, feel, and comport ourselves in conformity with the Cartesian way. We must disabuse our minds and bodies of the kind of assumptions that blind us to our active corporeal nature. We must learn to bodily resist taking the stance of a disembodied onlooker viewing reality through the narrow confines of the subject/object distinction. Besides exposing conceptual confusion and unexamined assumptions, another very powerful and effective way to free ourselves and enhance our manual therapy skills is to receive sessions of holistic manual therapy from a seasoned practitioner.

As we free ourselves at all levels, we come to depend less and less upon formulistic protocols and our perceptual skills become more and more accurate and uncanny. Practicing the three-step exercise presented in Chapter Seven will go a long way toward freeing and enhancing the necessary skills. Eventually, we find ourselves working more like a midwife participating in the birthing of order than a traffic cop. Our job is not to impose our somatic ideals on the body, but to allow the sentient body to express a more enhanced morphology. When therapy supports the body's own morphological imperative rather than one that is externally imposed, the body can more easily evolve into a new, more enhanced morphology. Maybe what results will match our somatic ideals and maybe it won't. But if the body renegotiates its verticality in the best way it can, it doesn't matter whether it matches our ideal or not because it will be functioning better. And better functioning will both create and support better structure.

To further illuminate and familiarize ourselves with the peculiarities of holistic seeing it would be helpful to look at the kinship between holistic and aesthetic perception by way of the felt-experiences of subjectivity and objectivity. When we look to the appreciation of beauty we see that it is a participatory form of perception. It creates a space that allows beauty to show itself. Aesthetic appreciation like holistic seeing does not require that we bodily shape ourselves into a detached onlooker separate from what is perceived. Instead, we allow what shows itself to shape our way of experiencing it in a participatory act of perception.

As a culture, we have lived the Cartesian worldview for so long and molded our perception with it so thoroughly that we have become very comfortable with living within the narrow confines of its experience of objectivity and subjectivity. It feels so familiar that it feels right to see the world through the eyes of a disembodied onlooker. But, if all we know is what shows itself in reflection to a detached bystander, we will be diminished by this orientation as will our perceptual skills. On the other hand, if our feeling-nature can freely open to a wide range and depth of experience, we will not be compelled to live this objectifying consciousness as the definitive expression of who and what we are. We also will not be tempted to go to the opposite extreme by rejecting this orientation altogether. We can also appreciate how the onlooker's orientation has its place, especially when involved in certain aspects of science. But, if we lack clarity about these experiences, we are more likely to take on a problematic way of narrowing down objective experience without noticing it. We will *feel* this narrowing of the objective world, and our relation to it is not only true but also the true way to feel when we are being objective. We then quite naturally live this narrowing of objectivity as the only way to feel true and the only true way to be. It feels orderly and right, not only because it feels familiar, but also because it feels the way things feel when they are grasped objectively as true.

Imagine an overly analytic person who adopts the orientation of the detached onlooker and feels this narrow form of objectivity as the primary way to be. Imagine further this person is asked to appreciate a beautiful work of art or witness a holistic assessment performed by an experienced manual therapist. He or she is likely to feel uneasy when hearing the requirement to openly participate with his or her whole being. This person no longer feels on solid ground because in comparison to how objectivity feels, this descent into subjectivity feels amorphous, lacking clear boundaries, and difficult to pin down. Felt-subjectivity soon comes to be associated with feelings of unclarity, amorphousness, and the lack of definitiveness. Whenever this person does not feel clear, he or she feels on the edge of an abyss of uncertainty and subjectivity. Clearly, subjectivity does not feel true the way objectivity feels true. In the Cartesian world, since what is not objective is necessarily subjective, the analytic, detached onlooker must conclude that the experience of beauty and the manual therapist's assessments are hopelessly subjective. What he or she mistakenly and prematurely feels as the lack of order makes him or her feel uneasy and unwilling to open-heartedly investigate it. It just does not feel right. So the person recoils from it and returns to the familiar well-defined confines of the narrowly objective.

The moment before he or she recoiled was the moment beauty began to show itself. Recall how Kant described in Chapter One the appreciation of beauty as the experience of orderliness that is created freely without concepts. Kant also recoiled. But his recoil was not because the fuzzy-headed ways of subjectivity made him nervous. It was because he wanted to believe that we could have knowledge of the external world without filtering it through our concepts. But his rationalistic Cartesian leanings offered no way to understand a non-conceptual grasp of being. Unlike our analytic onlooker, Kant stayed with his felt-subjectivity and investigated it rigorously. As we saw, Kant realized that beauty satisfies a deep primordial need for order. The pleasure we feel in the face of beauty is a deeply satisfying subjective experience. But it is a felt-subjectivity that is also universally true and possible for all cognitive beings. Since it rests upon the shared free play of the cognitive conditions that make knowledge possible, it has truth conditions. Because beauty appears without the need for concepts, the truth of aesthetic judgments cannot be easily and definitively stated. They can be profoundly felt, however. As a result, the orderliness of beauty has a felt depth of a different order than the conceptual order of the detached onlooker.

Generally speaking, a judgment is objective if it has truth conditions. For example, geology developed an objective test called the Moh scale to determine the hardness of rocks. You perform the test by rubbing two rocks together and the one not scratched is the harder of the two. Thus, we can say that the judgment "granite is harder than talc" has truth conditions and is objective.

For the most part, objectivity in the Cartesian worldview is narrowed down to the measurable. Since beauty cannot be measured, aesthetic judgments are not objective. But they are not merely subjective either if by subjective you mean that which is lacking truth conditions or universality. Lacking truth conditions means what is true for you is true for you but not necessarily true for me. Or to state this vacuous point differently, what is true for you could be false for me and both statements are true. Thus, there are really two kinds of subjectivity: the *merely subjective*, which lacks truth conditions, and the *universally subjective*, which has truth conditions. What I have been calling our feeling-nature is capable of revealing aspects of our world that are every bit as veridical as what is revealed to our senses. To most philosophically trained ears, the idea of a universal subjectivity sounds like an oxymoron because, like our analytic onlooker, they only recognize the merely subjective. But we now see that there is more to subjectivity and how our feeling-nature perceives its truths than most of us ever suspected.

When Kant turned his attention to aesthetic theory, he ceased recoiling because he realized a universal subjectivity in the appreciation of beauty. If our analytic, detached onlooker had stayed with the experience of subjectivity longer and hadn't recoiled before the merely subjective, he or she might have experienced a much grander and more profound sense of order than his or her narrowly defined conceptual order would permit.

Without embracing all the details of Kant's insights, we cannot help being impressed by what he tried to accomplish. At the risk of resting his philosophy on a possible oxymoron (universal subjectivity), Kant tried to make sense of a kind of judgment that was neither merely subjectively nor objectively measurable. In one bold stroke he changed the way we think about these matters. In pursuing his inquiry into the possibility of a universal subjectivity, he also opened up the inquiry into the possibility of a pre-conceptual comprehension of being. Whether we agree with Kant's solution or not, we can appreciate his attempt to elucidate and make sense of universal subjectivity. Because of the kinship between aesthetic experience and holistic assessments performed by manual therapists, his pursuit stimulates new insight, lends support to our inquiry, and gives us new ways to approach it.*

We typically do not experience how the onlooker stance turns the aesthetic into the anesthetic. If we are not sufficiently aware of how this subtle anesthetizing of our body happens, we will very likely not notice that we have become a detached onlooker who can only know and participate in the world by standing apart from it. More importantly, we will probably not recognize how our perceptual skills have suffered when we approach the world as a detached bystander disembodied onlooker. If we are not sufficiently attentive to this anesthetizing orientation, it can sap our perceptual vitality and become a major roadblock to holistic seeing.

In his or her premature retreat from the merely subjective to the narrowly objective, the detached onlooker naively and all too readily dismisses aesthetic judgments as merely subjective, while thoughtlessly declaring, "Beauty is in the mind of the beholder." We are now in a position to understand why the relegation of the aesthetic to the merely subjective is premature and naive. It rests upon the assumption, made questionable with the discovery of pre-reflective consciousness, that whatever is not objective is necessarily subjective. The discovery of the pre-reflective is the discovery of a third orientation of consciousness that is neither subjective nor objective, but is, rather, pre-subjective/pre-objective. As we will discover in Chapter Eleven there is an even deeper way of being with respect to all of this, which we can call the numinous and to which the pre-reflective is, metaphorically, a portal. We must let go of the onlooker's orientation if we are to understand and appreciate the depth of feeling-understanding that

---

*In fact, there are serious problems with Kant's way of securing truth conditions for aesthetic judgments. For a sustained critique of Kant's proof, see John Fisher and Jeffrey Maitland, "The Subjectivist Turn in Aesthetics: A Critical Analysis of Kant's Theory of Appreciation," *The Review of Metaphysics* 27, no. 4 (1974): 726–751. For an in-depth analysis of Kant's recoil and the solution he found in aesthetics, see also my "An Ontology of Appreciation: Kant's Aesthetics and the Problem of Metaphysics," *Journal of the British Society for Phenomenology* 13, no. 1 (January 1982): 45–68. Both articles are reprinted in Ruth Chadwick, ed., *Immanuel Kant: Critical Assessments* (Routledge, 1992)—a prestigious four-volume reference work of important writings on Kant.

holistic and aesthetic perception can call forth. For the manual therapist whose many ways of assessing are akin to aesthetic judgment, it is essential to know that they are not simply subjective fantasies. In comparison to the overly narrow felt-objectivity, holistic assessment and aesthetic perception often require a kind of speaking and description that is loose, image rich, and metaphorical.

Imagine you are standing before a painting by Rothko. As you read the description below, see if you can you feel the kinship between aesthetic experience and holistic assessments. We need to thoroughly familiarize ourselves with the language and experiences of both until they cease sounding like so much fuzzy-headed thinking instead of the insightful judgments they truly are. To allow the painting to show itself to you in its full sensuous presence, it helps if you know something about the history of painting in the twentieth century, especially color field painting, the emergence of abstract painting, and meta-art. Assisted by these aesthetic concepts, as you quietly contemplate the painting, you let the painting shape your way of seeing, and soon you begin to see it appear.

How might you describe what you are seeing? If you are to remain true to what is showing itself, you might be tempted to say something like the following: "After a few minutes alone with the Rothko I became aware of how the painting, which seemed empty of content, could yet avail itself of such a stunning depth of silence that it filled the room with a numinous presence." This way of speaking arises with participatory perception. It is not the reverie of subjectivity gone wild. It is characteristic of language that is attuned to the particular presencing of this way of painting. It speaks a language that is capable of disclosing how art is about the celebration and performance of its own origin. As such, this way of speaking is one of many accurate ways to describe the painting that is neither merely subjective nor narrowly objective, but can and often claims consensus.

Kant characterizes beauty as purposiveness without purpose. This is a shorthand way of saying that beauty exhibits a kind of orderliness that does not depend upon any concept of order. Thus, for example, Kant says that poetry occasions much thought but no definite thought. Predictably, the very features of aesthetic experience that make the analytic onlooker nervous are some of the same features that lovers of beauty cherish. With respect to the literary arts, it is why so many different interpretations are possible of a single work.

Hyper-reflexivity

Once free of the narrow confines of Descartes's understanding of subject and object, the implications for any form of therapy or counseling are straightforward: since cognitive and somatic order-thwarters can be so profoundly intertwined, giving up one's problematic worldview often requires being released from one's somatic conflicts and vice versa.

In his excellent explication of Merleau-Ponty's deconstruction of the concept of "consciousness" and "body," M. C. Dillon says, "Thought must be conceived as an extension of the body's perceptual powers, a development of reflexivity that is latent in perception ... [Merleau-Ponty] calls for a 'hyper-reflexivity' that thematizes and thereby neutralizes the distortions introduced by reflective thinking ... if reflection transforms the world by introducing an I, a thinking thing, then a further reflection can make itself aware of that fact and go on to understand that I as a product (rather than the condition) of thought.... The I of subjectivity, the reified agent of thought, comes into being through language, and the resulting grammatical habit becomes the basis of a philosophical prejudice. When the genesis of the I is understood, the I can return to the perceptual world and take up its proper abode in the lived body."[49]

But we need to be careful here. Two points require caution. Dillon's analysis of thought as an extension of the reflexivity latent in the perceptual powers of the lived body is an illuminating statement of how Merleau-Ponty understands the intertwining of thought and lived body. We also can immediately recognize in Merleau-Ponty's concept of hyper-reflexivity a useful tool for philosophical counseling or psychotherapy. The first note of caution concerns Dillon's problematic assumption that hyper-reflexivity is all that is required for overcoming conflicted and fixated forms of embodiment, or as he misleadingly says, the self's taking up its proper abode in the lived body. His assurance that hyper-reflexivity can overcome an alienated form of embodiment is also not borne out in the everyday work of holistic manual therapy, psychotherapy, or philosophical counseling. Overcoming alienation and finding our way back to healthier and less conflicted forms of embodiment is just not that simple. Secondly, every way you slice it, even as a metaphor, the notion of the "I taking up its abode in the lived body" thoroughly compromises the notion of the sentient body. The sentient body is not a fancy object or abode in which we somehow take up residence. The sentient body is not an object. Hence, it is not inhabitable. In part, it is a condition for inhabiting objects. Dillon's way of speaking simply falls back into the language of metaphysical dualism and all but resurrects it. Where would who or what inhabit this body-abode?

The alienation that is so prevalent in the modern world shows itself most clearly as conflicted and fixated forms of embodiment. Intentionality, as Merleau-Ponty says, is oriented space. It follows that a conflicted intentionality is a conflicted orientation in space that shows itself in the flesh, in conflicted ways of being-in-the-world, in conflicted forms of temporality, and in distorted thinking.*

I recall a depressed graduate student in philosophy who was dissociated from her feelings and collapsed body telling me, "You know, after years of therapy, I have come to understand that the philosophical theories to which I am most attracted and willing to defend arduously are the ones best suited to support my neurosis." Dillon's conclusion is too quick because it fails to appreciate how much of what we might call conflicted thinking, the distortions introduced by reflective thought, are anchored in perceivable distortions of the flesh and often serve to support defended and dysfunctional behavior. "Taking up the proper abode in the lived body" is a matter of living our embodied intentionality in a less conflicted, more

---

*For a discussion of conflicted forms of lived spatiality and lived temporality see my book *Spacious Body: Explorations in Somatic Ontology* (Berkeley: North Atlantic Books, 1995).

integrated way. Finding our way back to this way of being is almost never a simple matter of engaging in hyper-reflexivity. Often the return from alienation to integration is a rather lengthy and sometimes perilous journey requiring a variety of somatic, philosophical, and psychotherapeutic interventions, perhaps including years of meditation to fully comprehend the nature of the self. Clearly hyper-reflexivity can be a useful tool for psychotherapy, but by itself, it is hardly sufficient to show the way back to a less conflicted form of embodiment.

The Implications for Medicine in General

The claim that the body must be given its due in the context of all therapy would not be at all problematic to most somatic therapists. In fact, to those of us who deal with the body holistically, such an idea seems all but tautological. But I would guess that such a claim might not be so obvious to some philosophical counselors or psychotherapists. Experience shows that the body cannot be ignored in therapy or counseling of any kind. It is not uncommon to see clients who are unable to give up a conflicted worldview that sits at the core of their suffering because their tacit philosophical presuppositions were anchored in somatic fixations. If these somatic fixations are not released appropriately and in the right sequence, any attempt on the part of the psychotherapist to assist the client in seeing the way clear of these problematic philosophical presuppositions will meet with resistance or failure. Interventions can be completely ineffective and useless when the somatic aspect of the client's conflict is overlooked.

It is equally true that many somatic dysfunctions are tied to problematic worldviews. Just as some psychotherapists and philosophical counselors may not fully appreciate how a client's worldview can be rooted in somatic dysfunction, some somatic practitioners, whether they are Rolfers, osteopaths, chiropractors, or physical therapists, may not fully realize how profoundly a client's tacit or reflective worldview can influence the outcome of their therapeutic interventions. Even something as simple as a vertebra "being out of place," as it is often inappropriately described, can resist treatment—because it is connected to an unspoken but problematic worldview.

I am not suggesting that every somatic intervention must include philosophical counseling or psychotherapy any more than I am suggesting that every philosophical or psychological intervention must also include manipulating the body. But I am saying that understanding how a client's worldview can be an expression of conflicted somatic intentionality can be very useful to the psychotherapist or philosophical counselor. Knowing how to track the somatic aspects of how a client thinks about his or her world, for example, can make your work easier by showing where and where not to offer your philosophical probes or psychoanalytic interpretations.

This sort of understanding is especially critical once you realize that every form of medicine, therapy, or counseling ultimately must be considered holistic.* My claim that all therapy and medicine is, at bottom, holistic may sound somewhat excessive especially when you consider that the great majority of health care providers practice their art in a corrective rather than holistic way. But the realization that biological order is holistic entails that the most effective and appropriate treatment of our ills, aches and pains, and psychobiological problems must come from the holistic approach. Corrective strategies all approach the client in the same way. Specific problems are approached without concern for how they affect and are affected by the whole person and how he or she lives in his or her world. True, at times these specific problems can be handled quite appropriately without looking beyond the particular local somatic dysfunction or the particular conceptual or logical confusions of the client. But more times than not, a cognitive intervention will not be enough.

---

*For a more complete discussion of the differences between the corrective and holistic approaches see my discussion of the three paradigms of practice in my book *Spacious Body: Explorations in Somatic Ontology*, pages 145–152. For a study that shows that a holistic approach to chronic low back is more effective than the corrective approach, see John Cottingham and Jeffrey Maitland, "A Three-Paradigm Treatment Model Using Soft Tissue Mobilization and Guided Movement—Awareness Techniques for Patients with Chronic Low Back Pain," *The Journal of Orthopedic and Sports Physical Therapy* 26, no. 3 (1997): 155–167.

The following example is a good demonstration of how hyper-reflexivity and logic have little or no effect because they do not address the being of the whole person.

A manual therapist with some background in philosophical counseling was frustrated by a client who constantly appealed to Panglossian explanations as a way to avoid dealing with her problems. One day she said with her typical pseudo-cheeriness, "I think everything always works out for the best." "Good!" the counselor thought, "I can critique this philosophical position easily and show her some of her patterns of denial."

He began with an obvious distinction. "Some propositions are true or false and others are simply nonsense. If I were to say that the moon is made of green cheese, I would be making an empirical claim that, in principle, could be verified or falsified. Although it's a rather silly view, strictly speaking it is not nonsense, because we can verify the truth of my statement by going to the moon to see if it's made of green cheese." Barely taking enough time for a breath, he continued. "Your claim is neither true nor false because it is not an empirical one. We can see why by looking at an example. Suppose you have always wanted to own a Mercedes-Benz and you reach a point in your life when you realize it's not ever going to happen. In the face of not getting your Mercedes, you would have to say that it was for the best. But let's say the very next day some relative you hardly know dies and leaves you a Mercedes. Again, you would say that everything worked out for the best.

So moment by moment, every moment, no matter what happens, everything that happens is an example of working out for the best. Since no matter what happens—good, bad, or indifferent—everything that happens is an example of working out for the best. Unlike the claim that the moon is made of green cheese, your claim that everything works out for the best is not an empirical claim. We could go to the moon and find out whether it's made of green cheese. But since there are no imaginable conditions that could falsify your claim, your claim is vacuous. It is neither true nor false. It is quite simply non-sense." She looked at him for a while, then said, "Well, your logic is impeccable. But I like my theory better!"

As this example somewhat humorously demonstrates, neither hyper-reflexivity nor logic can be expected to make any difference if the whole person and the way she lives her world is not appropriately addressed. Also, because this philosophical counselor was frustrated by his client, he did not take the first step of the three-step process. Instead of stepping out of the way, he mildly abused her with logic.

Somatic and worldview fixations (order-thwarters) are dysfunctional whole patterns that usually involve the being of the whole person. They are rarely a local problem in the body or a specific confused concept. Because they are unified whole patterns themselves, they usually impel the whole person to adapt and reorganize around them. The concept of "fixation" is especially compelling when referring to psychological complexes and obsessions or to philosophical obsessions. However, since "fixation" implies a localized problem in the body that has no inherent connection to the whole, its use is less than ideal. The existence of such localized fixations in the body is pretty much a rarity. Therefore, I have been designating all fixations, whether they are found in our joints or worldviews, as "order-thwarters" as a way of calling attention to the fact that order-thwarters are unified whole patterns that are involved with and compromise the organization and freedom of the whole person.

Order-thwarters are patterns of perturbation that force the larger whole with which they are involved into new patterns of organization. A thwart at one level of our being tends to be a thwart at all levels. Since self-sensing constitutes part of our organismic identity and is distributed throughout the self-organizing pattern of our psychobiological nature, every system-wide thwart to our psychobiological organization also constitutes a possible thwart to our self-sensing. These thwarts to self-sensing compromise our freedom and make us less than what we could be. They adversely affect how we perceive the world, how we move, how we feel, and how we think. The more integrated and healthy our form of embodiment becomes, the freer we become from these order-thwarters. The freer we are from these thwarts to our existence, the clearer our self-sensing becomes and the freer we become. In fact, one of the indicators of a highly integrated person is a clear-minded imperturbability.

I want to emphasize the point that every system-wide thwart is a thwart to self-sensing as a way to underscore the fact that all medicine is necessarily holistic, even though most practitioners work in the second paradigm. Holism is not just about fixing parts, mobilizing joints, or engaging specific philosophical confusions. Holism is about freedom, about enhancing the being of the whole person, about allowing people to find themselves, about living richer and fuller lives, about feeling and being whole, about knowing who and what we are and how we fit into the larger whole of which we are an expression. It is about coming home.

No matter what kind of therapy we practice, we must always consider the whole person, his or her embodiment and way of living in his or her world. If we miss the impact of psychobiological order-thwarters or gravity and the environment on our clients, we are not seeing the whole of our clients' problems. As a result, our evaluation and treatment will be necessarily incomplete.

Understanding how thought and flesh intertwine is paramount to a successful outcome. In essence, every practitioner must become a holistic practitioner. If we can see clients holistically, then we can determine whether their problems can be approached from a purely corrective standpoint or from a holistic standpoint. But if we see clients from a corrective standpoint only, by necessity, we are not seeing the whole person. Many clinicians, especially the more experienced ones, often make these determinations intuitively. But only those who understand and are attentive to and truly understand the differences between the holistic and corrective approaches can clearly and responsibly determine the best approach for each client.

Conclusion

Our excursion into holism and manual therapy has yielded a rather surprising result—every form of medicine, from reflexology to brain surgery, is a form of holism. Furthermore, every dysfunction, every psychobiological confusion, every bodily woe is a holistic event relating holistically to the body as a whole. Order-thwarters are not isolated symptoms. They are also wholes. They are holistic dysfunctional patterns that compromise the whole body. To conceive of the body as an assemblage of parts and symptoms as isolated events is to fundamentally misunderstand the nature of biological order and how to intervene. As a result, the very same insurmountable assessment problems we discussed earlier face all forms of medicine when they are practiced in the second paradigm. Because second-paradigm practice is blind to holistic relationship, it is incomplete and runs the risk of being ineffective or harmful. Thus, each and every imaginable form of medicine or therapy must not only come to know and acknowledge that it is at bottom a holistic practice, but also learn to practice holistically and develop holistic eyes.

CHAPTER 11

Homecoming, Part II: Where You Always and Already Are

As we discovered in Chapter One, the experience of homecoming is the experience of freedom and beauty. The ability of the client to embody the freedom gained from receiving manual therapy is a good indicator that the client will hold on to the work. Not every client, however, can immediately grasp what has happened. In order to assist the client in cultivating and integrating the results, it is important for the practitioner to have a clear understanding of what freedom looks and feels like when it appears. To that end, we need to expand our understanding of homecoming to bring forth an aspect that has only been hinted at. On occasion, holistic manual therapy also seems to have the ability to open a person to what we might be tempted to call "the spiritual" dimension of life. In order to avoid steering our investigation into the problematic connotations associated with religion and religiosity, I will use the word "numinous" instead.

This chapter is meant to complete and deepen our understanding of homecoming. It offers glimpses into the numinous by displaying how activities as mundane as walking or running can serve as a portal to freedom and ends with examples of how manual therapy can assist clients in opening to the numinous.

Everything Moves

Everything moves. But we are self-movers who have no idea how it is that we move.

For the most part, we move through space, appropriating gravity, each movement flowing freely into the next, without ever giving it a thought. Generally, we do not think about the felt-experience of how we move; we just move when and where we want to. But have you ever wondered how you move your body, how you actually experience moving your body? To answer this question you must contemplate how you experience your movement as you live, breathe, and accomplish it. The question is asking for your point of view as the one who is moving, not for the point of view of an observer who is watching you move from the outside. Hence, for example, a neurological explanation of how you move is not an answer to the question.

We say with great confidence, "I move my body." What could be more self-evident than the knowledge that you are the mover of your body? Maybe your embodied self moves your body. If so, where is this embodied mover? How do I move my body if it is not a mere object? Try as I might, nowhere can I find the mover of this body. If I cannot find the mover of my body, how am I supposed to understand being embodied? Saying that I am embodied seems to suggest there was a time when I was out of my body, but now, thanks to my manual therapist, I am back in my body. But where and what is this "who" that slips so readily in and out of my body?

Upon first hearing these questions, we are frustrated by them and have little idea how to answer. But if you stay with your initial puzzlement, drop the demands of your thinking mind, and open yourself to really experiencing who moves and how you move, you could experience something truly remarkable. Like similar numinous questions, the answers have to do with our freedom—not as captured through words, but in direct experience.

How to Run Down a Mountain

In order to catch our first glimpse of how liberation can arise from the simple moment-to-moment free flow of everyday movement, let's look at a familiar experience of what athletes call "The Zone." The following description of running down a mountain comes from a graduate student. We will

148

be looking at three of his experiences with movement that occurred over a twelve-year period. The simplicity of his first experience may remind us of other similar kinds of experiences. The universality of these kinds of experiences also suggests that we are closer to realizing our freedom than we might have suspected. This description of running also provides us with just a hint of what is possible when we are able to transcend the confines of our limited I-am-self.

> The first time I saw the Colorado Rockies, I was an out-of-shape graduate student. A friend took me on a hike into the mountains. When we finally reached the top, my legs ached and my throat was on fire with my breath. After a short rest, we started down. To my surprise, my friend began running down the mountain. Being so uncertain on my feet and unsteady on the sliding gravel, I cautiously, and with what I thought was great care, placed one foot in front of the other, simultaneously probing each rock and pebble to make certain it would not slide. As a result, I repeatedly fell down. Finally, I gave up all caution and decided to follow my friend's example. With complete abandon and at the same time perfect precision, I ran down the mountain. When a rock slipped under my foot, I was able to leap in precisely the right direction so as to never fall or break my stride. Without there being time for calculation, my body knew exactly, with unerring awareness, what to do. When I reached the foothills, my legs no longer ached and my throat and lungs were no longer on fire. This abandoning of myself to movement was joyful and exhilarating.

Although this example is a pre-reflective and somewhat shallow experience of how freedom can arise in the mundane activity of running, it does give us a tantalizing taste of what is possible. Notice, the more the student reflected on how he was moving, the more he fell. His thinking self, his reflective self was too present. Finally, when he let go of all caution, he simultaneously let go of the confines of his self and became pre-reflective. He stopped thinking, and just ran. He was suddenly free of his reflective self—he was being run.

Looking more closely at the description, we also discover two ways of moving: one that is bound up with reflective thought and another that is pre-reflective and free of what my Zen teacher calls the "I-am-self" and its fixations. We will return to this distinction between reflective and pre-reflective thought later in this chapter.

Unfortunately, the most common understanding of how we move our body does little more than confuse an already confusing topic. It turns out to be much too narrowly conceived to grasp how liberation can arise from the simple moment-to-moment free flow of everyday movement. Since the most common answer is the most confused, we need to see through how it informs our thinking before we try to understand numinous movement.

I Will It to Move and It Moves

When asked, most people say that moving is simply a matter of willing yourself to move and then moving. This answer amounts to saying that all movement occurs in two phases: first, willing our body to move and then moving it. For the purposes of our discussion, we can call this answer the *I-will-it-to-move* theory. Notice how this answer seems to presuppose some version of metaphysical dualism where the body is at the bidding of the mind.

To see why this description does not apply to all movement and why it cannot grasp the appearance of freedom in moving, let's look at a simple example. Imagine we are eating a meal together. With your first bite you notice that your food is in need of salt. You have the idea for or, perhaps, just feel the urge for more salt. You ask me to pass the salt. My decision to pass the salt and the act of passing it occur simultaneously as one and the same movement. Without thinking about what I am doing, my eyes find the salt and my hand follows. Without giving it any thought whatsoever, without first willing my arm to move, my whole body participates in a fusion of flesh, feeling myself feeling, and intention as I simply flow with the urge to move my arm, grasp, and pass the salt, as if the series of intentions and action had become a single musical phrase. Without first willing your arm to move or thinking about it, or thinking about sensing your self sensing, your feeling-nature is saturated with the intention to receive the salt; your whole body participates in the movement of your arm. Like the notes in a musical phrase, your intention to receive the salt and the act of receiving it occur at the same time in the same felt movement.

As our example clearly demonstrates, our typical everyday way of moving does not take place in two phases. At the moment of receiving the salt, your self-sensing, reaching for it, and your intention to receive it are one and the same action. In actuality, intention, flesh, and movement are not separate. Rather, they are fused together in one unified action involving the entire body in our attempt to achieve a certain result. The decision to act and the resulting action occur at the same time in the same felt movement. In our everyday way of moving, there are not two phases; there is only one unified felt activity in which the will to move and the act of moving are two aspects of the same movement. Your self-sensing is always there implicitly and can be noticed at will.

As a way of adding authority to their view, some are tempted to dress up their account with a little neuroscience and claim, "First, I desire to move my arm. Then the brain and nervous system take over and move my body." Here is a more complicated but scientifically informed description: "If I wish to lift a glass to my mouth, I can conceive of this idea in my brain (perhaps stimulated by thirst, perhaps by my discomfort on a first date, it matters not), turn it into a code of dots and dashes, send this code down through the spine, out through the brachial plexus, and down to my arm. At the neuromuscular junction, the message is decoded into meaning—and the relevant muscles contract according to the coded sequence."[50]

Although more scientifically informed, this sort of description utterly fails to capture our experience. No one experiences moving his or her arm this way. This description of coding and decoding into movement is theory masquerading as a description of experience. The first thing to notice is that the description conflates first-person experience with third-person experience. In the laboratory, the kinesiologist is not describing your experience of movement as you feel and live it. The explanation of neural activity in terms of decoding dots and dashes is not a first-person description. It is rather a third-person description made by an onlooker. Once again, we see Descartes's influence at work. Although the details are different because the science is more evolved, we see the same conflation of experience (first-person experience) and causal explanation (third-person account) that we first encountered in Chapter Six.

In the end, no matter how much detail you fill in about how the brain and nervous system take over, you cannot escape the fact that this answer verges on being a form of metaphysical dualism that is a slightly more complicated variation of the I-will-it-to-move theory we just looked at. Throwing a little science into the mix adds nothing to its explanatory power because the theory is based on the very same one-sided description. If you fail to see the conflation, mixing up lived experience with scientific explanation may appear to give your descriptions more authority than they deserve.

Not convinced by the I-will-it-to-move answer but unable to say why, many people defiantly throw their hands up and declare, "I just move!" While such a response is not really an answer, it often expresses the suspicion that there is more to moving than is stated by the I-will-it-to-move description and the frustration that comes from trying to describe a whole body orientation and movement in which desire, intention, flesh, and feeling are somehow fused into an inseparable unity.

The I-will-it-to-move view probably seems suspicious to many because it also suffers from the unspoken assumptions of metaphysical dualism: mind and body are two separate and distinct entities and that moving our body can be understood on the model of moving an object. Nothing could be further from the truth. For example, picking up our arm is nothing like picking up a shovel. It does not even feel remotely like picking up a shovel. When we move our arm, we do not experience ourselves as picking up and moving a separate isolated object. Rather, our entire body participates in the movement of our arm, which is experienced as both the fulfillment and manifestation of our desire and intention. We feel our arm move in such a way that it orients our whole body in a unified action saturated with the intention to accomplish something. It is not a cognitive act. Rather, it is an example of lived experience that is lived as felt. We clearly do not experience our arm as an isolated mere thing that we mysteriously sling into moving by means of our will. I do not feel the shovel as an aspect of me or in any way how I feel myself to be. The movement of my arm is the movement of my fleshy intention flowing and leading the way as one felt unified pre-reflective action in which I bodily orient toward accomplishing something. I know where I am in space because I feel where I am. Wielding a shovel in space does not feel the way I experience using my arm in space. Poetically speaking, such free, unencumbered movement is like air becoming form. Movement is the visible activity of mind.

But when all is said and done, the most telling argument against the I-will-it-to-move description comes from the simple recognition that it ignores our typical felt-experience. Our experience shows us, again and again, that the way we typically move minute-to-minute is not a matter of first willing our body or some part of our body, as if it were a separate object, to move and then moving it. Our sentient body is not a mere thing, and its movement clearly does not always involve two distinct phases: an act of will and then an action that follows. Just think how peculiar we would look if walking were dominated by having to will each step to move before moving it and then moving it. We would look like some sort of herky-jerky marionette. Or perhaps an even better example is Jacques Tati's lovable character, Mr. Hulot, whose stop-and-go, haltingly indecisive walking seems to go in multiple directions at once, as if he were being driven by seemingly contradictory intentions.

Thinking about Moving

Normally, our minute-to-minute ways of moving are performed as a seamless fusion of intention and flesh where the desire to move and the resulting act is one and the same movement of the sentient body, and where each movement flows freely into the next. This way of moving only happens when we are not attending to it or not trying to make ourselves move in new ways. The exquisite free flow of movement disappears the minute you think about it. Furthermore, attending to our movement while moving is usually an indication that something is wrong or that a movement is new to us. Consider how much we have to think about what we are going to do before we do it when we are recovering from injury or learning a new dance step.

Thus, the kinds of movements partially captured by the I-will-it-to-move theory are, for the most part, performance difficulties that require our thinking about them before moving. What the I-will-it-to-move description brings to light is that movements that involve performance difficulties have two phases. The first phase is about the intention or desire to move in a new way, and it usually involves planning and thinking about how we are going to move. Although there is a tendency to construe the first phase as the cause of movement, a moment's reflection reveals that it is actually the reason for it. The second phase is practicing and trying to move in the new way.

Oddly, even though the moment-to-moment, free flow of one movement into another is our most common experience of movement and the one closest to us, it is also the movement we have the most trouble recognizing and describing. Part of the reason we have trouble getting a handle on it is that it is the kind of movement that only appears when we are not attending to it. You cannot think about this kind of movement and do it. You can only live it. The moment we attend to it, it disappears and becomes an object of scrutiny for reflective thought, and the more we think about it, the less free our movement becomes. Unlike performance difficulties such as learning how to dance or walk after an injury that requires thinking about how we are going to move, the ubiquitous free flow of movement that fills our days requires just the opposite—that we do not think about it. For the most part, however, we are only vaguely aware of the unified free flow of the whole body in movement. As a result, we tend to miss just how exquisite our moment-to-moment flow of movement can be and how much of our days are alive with it.

It's Not Unconscious Either

Interestingly, our rather circuitous investigation into the experience of self-movement has revealed two ways of moving. One way requires thinking about how we are going to move before we actually move, and the other more ubiquitous way of moving occurs in the absence of reflective thought. The observation that our free minute-to-minute movement does not involve thinking suggests to some that it is unconscious. But as it turns out, the reflective/pre-reflective distinction from the discipline of phenomenology is much more suited to the job of understanding these two forms of movement.

Consider your experience when you are completely engaged in and given over to some activity, say, playing a piece of music or playing a close game of basketball. If your musical performance is at all inspired, you will not be thinking about your performance. There will be no "you" wondering about how you are doing. The same is true if you are giving your all in a basketball game. Even though you're not thinking, you are consciously participating with what is unfolding. During the musical performance, you become one with the music as it pre-reflectively flows through you. Only later, when the performance is over do you think about it. When the music flows through you unencumbered by thinking, your experience is pre-reflective. When you step out of the flow of lived experience and think about various aspects of your performance, your experience is reflective.

Recall the graduate student's experience of running down the mountain. The more he thought about where to place his feet and how to avoid falling, the more he fell. He was reflecting too much on his experience. But the moment he gave up trying to think himself down the mountain, he found himself pre-reflectively running free. As professional athletes like to say, he was in the zone.

Pre-reflective experience is both pre-subjective and pre-objective. In the process of moving toward reflection, we separate ourselves from lived experience, and the participatory understanding of pre-reflection falls apart into the subject and object. Notice that pre-reflective experience is a form of consciousness and orientation of the sentient body that is neither subjective nor objective. The pre-reflective/reflective distinction does not just apply to what we call mind. Properly considered, it applies to the orientation of our whole being, sentient body and all.

The pre-reflective/reflective distinction is a philosophical distinction. By virtue of being the broader distinction, it includes the psychological distinction between the conscious and unconscious. The unconscious is that aspect of our pre-reflective experience that we, either through self-deception or lack of interpretive skill, misinterpret to ourselves and others in reflection.

At this point in our discussion, it is probably already clear how the pre-reflective/reflective distinction applies to our two forms of movement. Our ubiquitous experience of the free flow of moment-to-moment movement is properly understood as a pre-reflective experience. The two-phased movement that we uncovered through investigating performance difficulties is a clear example of reflective experience.

Who Moves?

Many of us spend so much of our days thinking about this and that that we completely miss the flow of pre-reflective moment-to-moment freedom of movement that is, for the most part, our constant experience. If you dig yet deeper into the kind of movement that does not involve thinking, you will also discover that there is no enduring self or entity that moves your body. As we make our way through the world dealing with the obstacles and difficulties along the way, nothing seems more certain than I am the mover of my body. But if you try to locate the mover of your body, you cannot find it. Not only that, since your body is not an object, figuring out what you are doing when you move it also has its challenges. The more we consider this question about who moves our body, the more ridiculous it seems. How can it be that there is no self that moves my body when it is so obvious that I am the mover of my body? When I look for it, the self I thought myself to be has no shape, weight, or place to be. But who is the mover, after all, if not me?

Even when faced with the inability to find a continuous self-subsisting self, the claim that there is no continuous self that moves our body still seems wildly counterintuitive. But look again. Nowhere in your pre-reflective experience of the free flow of moment-to-moment movement do you find a continuous self-entity that moves your body. There is just the pre-reflective orientation of your sentient body, fully aware, assessing and negotiating its way through the obstacles, joys, and difficulties of its world. There is no separate self-subsisting self doing the movement. There is only your active sentient body, where intention and flesh are inseparable, and where the intention to move and the act of moving are one and the same movement.

Our movement mostly occurs at a pre-reflective level where the intention to move and the actual movement are experienced as one and the same action. At the pre-reflective level there is no reflective self in play. There is only just pre-reflectively conscious, intelligent, purposeful moving. Later when you think about or report on what you were pre-reflectively doing, you introject a self into your experience. You say, "I moved," and falsely believe your reflective self was there all along. But clearly, a reflective self cannot be present in pre-reflective movement.

Your self is neither continuous nor any kind of entity. Other than where your sentient body is, your self has no specific location. There is no internal control center where it sits and moves your body. Instead, your body is saturated with mind and intention. Mind and body are not mutually exclusive, incommensurable ontological kinds. They are implicated in each other. Even at the pre-reflective level your bodily orientation and movement are infused with an awareness of your surroundings as you make your way through our shared world.

To avoid confusion one last distinction should be made before we leave this discussion of self. Consider more carefully your pre-reflective experience and notice that there is a subtle sense of unity that is present in your experience. It is not an entity and it is not continuous. It is a felt-sense of bodily unity, a felt-sense that we rarely properly identify and often confuse with a sense of self. But the denial of the existence of self is not a denial of the sense of bodily unity in activity or repose. Notice too that a felt-sense of bodily unity is not the sort of phenomenon that could move a body.

Thus, the answer to the question "Who moves?" becomes more transparent. If you mean by "self" a continuous self-subsisting entity, then there is no such thing that moves our body. If you mean by "self" the felt-sense of bodily unity, a felt-sense is not a self-entity and it also comes and goes. Lastly, if all you mean by self is the non-continuous sense of identity that only appears when we reflect on our experience, then the manifestation of a reflective self when we are having performance difficulties or thinking about our movement is how self primarily appears in movement. Otherwise, there is very little in the way of a reflective self involved in moving our sentient body.

We easily recognize how we structure our day-to-day activities by means of reflective thought, but we are mostly oblivious to the role the pre-reflective plays in our day-to-day activities. As a result, we almost entirely overlook the kind of bodily intelligence that is always at work in our daily life. Because we think of our body as a fancy object that we inhabit, the idea of a thinking body or sentient body never occurs to us. But our sentient body is capable of assessing, negotiating, and making its way through the world without engaging in reflective thought or presupposing a self-entity. When all is said and done, you are not other than your body. And, of course, it is you who moves your body—it's just not by means of a self-entity or any kind of continuous self.

KABOOM!

With the recognition that there is no self-entity moving our body, we seem to have arrived at a fundamental insight of Buddhism concerning the existence of the self. But let's look more closely. The Buddha's discovery actually goes to the very origin of self and world and, hence, to the origin of the pre-reflective and the reflective. As a result, pre-reflective experience and the Buddha's experience cannot be the same. But, as we are about to see, sometimes something as simple as pre-reflective walking can transform itself into a numinous experience of the source, thus demonstrating how pre-reflective activity can be a gateway to freedom.

Whether we realize it or not, we and the totality of what is are always returning to zero, dissolving into oneness, and being reborn. Imagine you are leisurely walking down the street. Suddenly and without warning, a car backfires behind you. KABOOM! For an instant, you and the kaboom, time and space, subject and object become one. At zero, there is no self in place to record the passage of time. There is only unity and unencumbered love. Then, just as suddenly as everything became one, your self reappears and you begin thinking about what just happened. "Oh man! I thought that was a gun being fired."

In the same way you died and resurrected with kaboom, throughout your day, in the very first moment of meeting the things and people of your world, you instantly become one with them and then just as quickly separate. When you were strolling down the street, you were sometimes orienting pre-reflectively and sometimes reflectively. But when the car backfired, all sense of self, identity, as well as your pre-reflective world simply disappeared in oneness and love. Because we are not looking for this activity and it occurs so quickly, we usually miss it.

Whether we realize it or not, it is the same when we first meet anything. For example, in the very first moment you see a tree, you and the tree become one. As result, there is no distance and no difference between you and the tree, and there is no pre-reflective or reflective orientation. But, in the next instant when your self resurrects commenting on the magnificence of the tree, a distance and a difference manifests between you and the tree. Even when you are looking at the tree pre-reflectively, a sense of a distance and a difference still exists between you and the tree. But when we return to zero, we are completely one with the tree, the reflective and pre-reflective have disappeared, and there is neither distance nor difference.

Unfortunately, we all too easily lose track of how we become one with everything and mistakenly believe that our self is an enduring entity that is the essence, center, and foundation of what we are. Just as we mistakenly perceive our self to be an entity having duration, we also mistakenly perceive our body and all existing things as having a self-subsisting nature that endures.

Why Did Bodhidarma Walk to China?

When our everyday pre-reflective movement is practiced as a form of meditation, it can grant us access to the numinous. Since Zen Buddhism is a non-dogmatic, body-oriented, practice-based discipline that emphasizes firsthand experiential verifiability, it is an ideal practice for studying walking meditation. Zen is an intense course of study, involving a number of practices, including long hours of meditation, punctuated with walking meditation (known as kinhin in Japanese Zen).

The practice of Zen is not designed to provide the practitioner with a comforting set of beliefs or an alternative explanation of the nature of reality. Rather, it is designed to offer an *alternative to explanation* by allowing the practitioner to solve the riddle of life based on his or her own direct experience of reality.* In a sense, the practitioner wakes up to the way things truly are and his or her place in all of this.

There are many practical benefits that come from walking meditation. Zen retreats are usually seven days long often beginning at three o'clock in the morning and ending around nine or ten o'clock at night. After a few days of this daunting schedule your legs, back, and other structures can start to ache, spasm, or fixate. Walking can help alleviate or ameliorate these kinds of problems. It also can help keep the joints of the low back (lumbar spine and sacroiliac joints) mobile and free of pain. But one of the more important purposes of walking meditation is to bring the experience of sitting meditation into action and the numinous into movement.

---

*The idea of providing an alternative to explanation comes from Henri Bortoft's explication of Goethe's qualitative science of nature. I appropriated his phrase in order to make an important point about the nature of Zen practice. In so doing, I may have changed its original meaning. See *The Wholeness of Nature: Goethe's Way toward a Science of Conscious Participation in Nature.* (New York: Lindisfarne Press, 1996).

As a way to take our second tentative step toward understanding how freedom can manifest through walking, let's look at how it showed up five years later for our intrepid graduate student. He had earned his PhD after a period of arduous study and then became a Zen student. His second experience of walking meditation brings us closer to the numinous than his first experience of running down the mountain.

ZEN WALKING

After twenty-five hours of travel and a sleepless plane flight, I arrived in Japan at seven o'clock in the morning dead tired. My good friend was there to meet me. We had to run errands all over Tokyo and arrived at my friend's house late that night. I was so depleted after traveling that I could not form words with my mouth anymore. I fell in bed totally exhausted.

We rested the next day and on the following day set off for my first Zen retreat. I was still quite exhausted from my arduous journey and somewhat worried by the thought of getting up at three o'clock in the morning for seven days. The retreat turned out to be more difficult than I had ever imagined possible. The pain in my legs from sitting cross-legged was intense and it was all I could do to stay awake.

Even walking meditation was difficult for me. This particular temple supplied all the participants with straw sandals that we were required to wear during walking meditation and walking in the temple. Unfortunately for me, the largest pair were half the size of my foot. Walking in them was quite painful and awkward. As a result, I had trouble staying in step with the kinhin line. Exhausted and in pain, I kept at it.

On the morning of the third day during walking meditation, quietly and without warning, something shifted in me. Up until that moment I felt as if I were confined in a completely oppressive space, burdened with numerous aches and pains and emotional traumas and so exhausted that I could barely see straight. Then, suddenly I was wide awake, feeling as though I were completely at home, unburdened and alive, full of peaceful clarity, and luxuriating in the expansiveness of the softest, most spacious, heartfelt energy imaginable. I felt free for the first time in my life. My mind was like the great expanse of the sky. My consciousness was no longer dominated by thinking. There was no me doing the walking. It was if something much vaster had taken over and was doing the walking. I was enraptured by the mere act of walking. I was not walking—I was being walked. How could I have passed over this way of walking in my day-to-day life? I remembered similar experiences when jogging. But that was nothing compared to the freedom I was experiencing now.

Walking free of the fixations of my self brought with it the most delicious sense of freedom I had ever experienced. Moment by moment, step by step, the in-here and the out-there turned out to be the same here. Step after step I was being walked free of all cares and troubles at every level of my being. I felt clear and bright, as if my entire being had undergone a profound cleaning, and was subsequently filled with the greatest sense of freedom imaginable. Instead of resting during the breaks, I spent every remaining rest period in walking meditation, allowing myself to be carried away by being walked. Beauty was now underfoot wherever I walked, and wherever I walked my heart sang.

His second experience of the numinous went a little deeper and dramatically demonstrated how the mundane activity of walking can be transformed into a numinous experience of freedom. He had the advantage of beginning his retreat exhausted, and at the end of the rope. The retreat pushed him beyond his limits, he held on until he couldn't any longer, and then he simply let go and surrendered his limited human perspective and came home.

It is possible to wake up to the wonder of what is always happening—provided you are willing to surrender to your everyday way of walking so completely that you perceive how the true state of affairs comes to presence in the ordinary. You will not find this freedom in pre-reflective action alone. But as we have repeatedly seen, pre-reflective action can be a gateway to the numinous. If you give yourself over completely to pre-reflective action, in the simple act of walking you can know the boundless freedom and unencumbered love that appears when you become one with the numinous activity of the source. In ways we do not fully understand, similar awakenings to how things really stand can occur through holistic manual therapy.

When somebody wakes up to the way things truly are and finds his or her place in all of this, he or she develops the ability to know the love that permeates the cosmos. He or she comes to know the activity of the source not because he or she believes it or has a theory about it, but because of the direct experience of it. This kind of knowing sets one free. As a result of it, everyday life becomes more and more like a homecoming as he or she manifests more and more profoundly the qualities of being embodied.

Clients who embody their freedom in this way exhibit similar qualities. They are organized around the vertical and horizontal spatiotemporal fields. They are able to meet the world with full presence and humor. Typically, they move with grace, ease, and purpose. Even if they are injured or handicapped, they are easy with themselves and know who they are. Their fluid coordinated movement is an expression of being grounded and uplifted, and integrated in gravity. Many such clients also develop and manifest a compassionate clear-minded imperturbability.

Because manual therapy is capable of removing the thorns of the flesh and putting the whole person right with his or her environment, it is capable of opening some people to the numinous. To illustrate this possibility, let's look at the results of a couple of different sessions of manual therapy. Our first example comes from our PhD Zen student when he was in the process of being Rolfed. One evening after a magnificent Colorado blizzard he received a session of manual therapy from a very creative Rolf movement practitioner and Rolfer.

TROMPING IN THE SNOW

As soon as the session started, my Rolfer noticed something odd in my legs, especially in my feet—something about not contacting the Earth. Using her considerable manipulative skills combined with exquisite attention to my breathing, she managed to get my legs to where they supported my body with an ease that seemed absolutely effortless. "Whose legs are these?" I thought to myself. And then suddenly I noticed my feet. They felt wonderful, like two pads softly connecting into the Earth, giving me the sense of being supported and energized by forces unseen, but palpable. I am new to Rolfing, so I am not sure what she did and how she did it. But by the time she was halfway through the session I was spacious and alive: standing tall, happy, and grounded. She did not just get me aligned in gravity, she brought me in tune with my surroundings. Once again I was experiencing the familiar freedom, lightness, and open heart that I felt running down the mountain and doing walking meditation.

I left the session feeling washed clean, free of my burdens, and in love with everything. The blizzard had abated but the amount of snow it dumped was tremendous. I was so thrilled with how my legs and feet felt as I walked through the deep snow that I continued tromping, running, falling down, and jumping for hours, all the while laughing. I woke the next morning debilitated by sore muscles and stiffness. I had really overdone it. But surprisingly I was still happy and my heart was still open. Oh yeah . . . I almost forgot my feet, my wonderful feet . . . What a gift!

These last two examples show us yet another side.

PETER: BEING HERE

Peter was a tall, lanky, and rather slender man. He was well spoken and obviously highly educated. He was concerned with his poor posture and was hoping that advanced Rolfing would make a difference. Although he did not have full-blown scoliosis, his spine did exhibit a number of aberrant patterns and curvatures that also affected the shape of his rib cage. These shapes, in turn, expressed the way he stood and balanced in gravity as well as how he oriented toward and was solicited by his world. As I worked with him he told me his story: an odyssey of self-discovery and waking up to a newfound sense of belonging. What follows is our collaborative attempt to tell his story as accurately as we can.

Peter sought my services on the heels of his fifty-fifth birthday. His experience with various forms of manual therapy and psychoanalysis spanned over four decades comprising two distinct phases. The first phase began with receiving the traditional ten-session protocol of Rolfing when he was an undergraduate at the University of Colorado during the late 1970s. The second phase began when he received his first session with me in 2009. Since that time he has received around twenty sessions from me. He was passionate about Rolfing and his enthusiasm for it never waned.

After graduating from college he experienced a severe upheaval in his personal life. He was in bad shape financially and his life stagnated uncontrollably as he gave into wallowing in a life without direction. Between the two phases, he went through a very dark and difficult time. During this long "dark night of the soul," he could only afford to get Rolfed now and then. Over time, it slowly dawned on him that his self-defeating nihilistic worldview, stagnation, lack of direction, and lack of resources were all connected to his inability to meet his world. To a Rolfer's eyes these issues could be seen in his sentient body. His body's way of shaping his lack of integration showed up in how he psychobiologically withdrew from a world he found overwhelming and could not understand.

Peter was painfully aware of how his postural imbalance, aberrant patterns of movement, dysfunctional childhood, and repression all contributed to his pervasive ontological insecurity and fundamental ambivalence toward being embodied. He was also convinced that his lifelong lack of balance and coordinated movement inclined him toward seclusion and introspection, which was exacerbated in later childhood by excessive weight gain.

He first encountered Rolfing in the hothouse ferment of self-realization that characterized Boulder during the late 70s. Peter painfully recalled his ceaseless endeavor to maintain a well-adjusted façade despite an ongoing sense of alienation and estrangement from his body and world. At the end of the day, he could neither study nor party authentically. After graduation he lapsed into the lifestyle of a perennial graduate student. He was offered a number of fellowships that he deferred because of a lack of confidence in his ability to function outside his accustomed habitat. He toiled as an editorial assistant while immersing himself in psychoanalysis, analytic psychology, and Eastern philosophy, especially Buddhism. He participated in various self-styled meditation groups, which often created considerable psychic conflict in him. Under the guise of surrendering his ego, one of his meditation teachers demanded that he give up all his autonomy and follow his teacher without question. For five or six more years he continued to search for a spiritual path that made sense to him, but to no avail. After an aborted start in yet another graduate program, he finally settled into a graduate program at a high-ranking university. For nearly a decade he unsuccessfully tried to balance coursework while pursuing an alternative career in academic administration.

Peter's first Rolfer was an angry anti-intellectual and professed champion of the counterculture who made no effort to disguise his contempt for Peter's intellectual endeavors. As Peter said, "It is ironic that a practitioner of somatic therapy could so insidiously saddle a client with guilt, ambivalence, and inhibition. . . ." But saddle him he did and despite himself Peter introjected the Rolfer's negativity. Peter carried the introjection for the intervening years until his first session with me. When Peter told me about his first Rolfing session, I immediately worked to disabuse him of it. When he was finally free of all the negativity his Rolfer left him with, he was immediately aware of a positive change in his posture. As a last thought, I added, "You know, anti-intellectualism is an incoherent point of view. An anti-intellectual is an intellectual who turns his intellect against the intellect."

Sometime after he experienced work from the anti-intellectual therapist, he tried a single session with another manual therapist who left Peter so emotionally vulnerable that he sobbed and convulsed uncontrollably for hours on end over a period lasting more than a week. Looking for just a single word of reassurance that he was going to be all right, or some explanation of what was happening to him, he repeatedly tried to contact the manual therapist by phone only to be rebuffed.

Peter reports that the advanced Rolfing he has received from me has proven to be life-changing. Without any intent of hyperbole he reports that the new and improved sense of symmetry, coordination, and poise he experiences following each session is a "dream come true." Even after just the first session he could feel himself being liberated from the bodily constraints and dysfunctional patterns that had encumbered his engagement with the world and hampered his most basic human impulses to participate in meaningful interpersonal relationships. He was excited to discover that he finally had the capacity to socialize without effort—"to hang out" and be a "regular guy" among friends and colleagues as he put it. Each successive session further consolidated his sense of balance and order. This consolidation made it increasingly possible for him to have more effortless social interactions.

Improved integration has brought even more fluidity, ease, and confidence to Peter's movement. He reports experiencing a new sense of vigor, which brings with it the enjoyment of competing with others without the fear of "falling apart." He indicates that he is increasingly more likely to initiate projects and tasks that require physical exertion and far less likely to abandon them if they become difficult to manage.

He reports that his ability to extrapolate from existing knowledge and engage in sustained conversation—to "think on his feet"—has improved dramatically while a new capacity for prolonged focus and concentration has brought more nuance and depth to his scholarship. He is more likely to "stand his ground" in the face of disagreement and better able to negotiate complex interpersonal interactions. He has become deft at dodging unnecessary conflict. He procrastinates less and finds that he accomplishes simple tasks without hesitation or excessive deliberation. He feels more spontaneous and creative and is better able to multitask, which he likens to expanded broadband access. He even reports that his sense of humor has improved and that he sleeps better. He has also been able to realize the kind of job he has always wanted. As a result, his professional career is no longer in a hopeless death spiral.

The extent of the improvement Peter reports in physical, psychological, cognitive, emotional, and spiritual functionality is a stunning testimony to the transformational power of holistic manual therapy, what we might metaphorically call its inherent alchemical potential to induce meta-somatosis, the enhancement of the whole person through the enhancement of the lived body.

Here is the last example.

THE TUNNEL OF LIGHT

In my case, I came to Rolfing with a body that had endured a bad marriage, a resentment-filled divorce, several career crises, and a near-fatal auto accident seven years prior. The body spoke eloquently of these things by a chronic sinus condition, nagging back aches, and an occasional muscle spasm across the shoulders. On a more subtle level, there was also a persistent inability to swallow, fleeting anxiety flutters in the region of the heart, and annoyingly regular colds. Despite all of this, I held the belief that I was quite healthy: in other words, I simply wasn't listening to my body. The voice it had fell on deaf ears. My intellect routinely overrode the messages of imbalance my body communicated.

In retrospect, I have come to realize that I, like so many of my contemporaries, did not know my body, did not fully trust it, and, most certainly, did not live in it. I was almost entirely an intellect, residing in a system that I placed in low regard. The body was devalued and dishonored by neglect.

Each person's body, it seems, contains an emotional blueprint and a spiritual map for that lifetime. Certain goals and principles are expressed in the physical form taken and shaped over time. To work with the body, then, is to touch the past, the present, and the future simultaneously. Memories of the life that was and dreams of that yet to come dance wistfully on the fingertips of the Rolfer. At times, waves of emotions swirl and abound as the tissue is touched and changed. In the hands of the Rolfer lies the Universe, contained in the body of a single human being. Each cell beats with a life force composed of energy, rhythm, and sensation. Such work is sacred, as holy as the miracles of scripture and history recorded in the days of the Ancients. For here, in this body, resides God, and Spirit, and Oneness.

I was unprepared for that knowledge when, in one lengthy session, I witnessed a white shaft, tube-like, a tunnel of light arising from within me and emerging out of my head, expanding farther and farther beyond me. It drifted higher and higher, seemingly reaching for the sky, all the while stretching effortlessly from my physical self, connecting me to the vast unseen. I dubbed it my "holy spirit," and felt such peace and elation as I had ever felt. My sense, then and now, is that it was a unified vision arising spontaneously from the release of energy, previously blocked from expression. Held trapped in a body harnessed with trauma and memories, this knowledge was kept prisoner in my body, locked away from my awareness. Once released, it beat a gentle pulsation, and danced a joyful, soaring dance into timelessness. With that vision has come a sense of the unity and grace of our reality, and lifetimes, and existences. With that vision has gone the fear and aching anxiety of the Void, for now purposefulness is known and embraced.

The Rolfer acts as a conduit for the spirit in body so that it might align itself with the life path and goal of the person being Rolfed. Restoring the means of expression so that energies might flow freely, cutting away restrictive ties, loosening tight restraints on a muscular level, he or she works to create lightness. This lightness I feel on multiple levels: in my physical sense as I move, in my emotions as I feel graced by the depths of my feeling states, and, spiritually, as I capture a vision of the truer reality of my own world of experience. I am light, lighter, and lightness itself.

Rolfing is a transformative process; I have been changed by the experience. Not only do I sense my world more acutely, but I envision more elaborately as well. I have an intensified feeling about such things as honesty and deception. I tolerate less easily the day-to-day idiotic dances of illusion most of us endure for sheer survival. I suspect that I will leave behind the willingness to "make do" and replace it with a desire to expand the self that I now know to be truly limitless!

I believe that the mind exists throughout the body; we think with our whole selves, not just in the brain. We are an energy field, a living, breathing Universe. The wonder of it fills me with a sense of the miraculous. I live my body now with a fascination born of new insights. I revere the holistic human being I am with a grateful heart; I have found a transcendent self only hinted at in earlier living.

The future unfolds itself within me; the past resides more amicably now with my present self. Integration is continuing and my spirit self has married my mind and heart; it is a joyful union![51]

Conclusion

Our excursion into the numinous showed us the difference between the pre-reflective and the numinous. When our walking is unencumbered and pre-reflective, the freedom we experience seems similar to what we experience in homecoming. But it only seems so. Notice, our pre-reflective consciousness can be so swamped with feeling that it obscures the potential for freedom that lives in the heart of our everyday ways of moving. To make the point with an extreme example, consider the plight of a paranoid person who is condemned to feeling paranoia pre-reflectively. The numinous is not limited to the pre-reflective. It is prior to the pre-reflective/reflective distinction. And it cannot be overwhelmed.

Whether we walk by ourselves or with others, whether in the city or hiking a mountain trail, instead of just being walked, we find ourselves occupied with endless concerns, ideas, plans, worries, anticipations, and random thoughts. We are often so caught up by the flow of thoughts and concerns that we barely even register the fact that we are moving with utter freedom as each movement flows unencumbered into the next. Whether we realize it or not, moment by moment, one step after another, we are appearing and disappearing, dying and resurrecting with the totality of what is in the free flow of one movement into another.

CHAPTER 12

The Poetics of Manual Therapy

After all this discussion about the practice, philosophy, and meta-theory of manual therapy, perhaps it would be useful and informative to spend this last chapter looking at the experience of the manual therapist when doing his or her work. It goes without saying that manual therapists want to help people, to give them back their functionality, to relieve their pain, and when it is appropriate in some cases, perhaps provide a portal to the numinous. But the question I am asking is about what it is like for the manual therapist when he or she performs his or her work. When you see a skilled manual therapist in love with his or her work, what is his or her experience of doing the work? What does it mean *to get* the work of manual therapy?

Getting It

When you truly *get* something, your sentient body *gets* it. Analogous to the way your whole body and mind are seized with laughter when you get a joke, or are moved to tears when you hear an inspired performance of music, the wholeness of who you are is seized with understanding when you get manual therapy. If your body is not affected in any way, you are probably not getting it. When you get being a manual therapist, you are also seized with understanding—the practical bodily know-how to transform lives by transforming bodies. Your sentient body is possessed of an uncanny know-how that fills you with a profound sense of freedom and the sense that something greater is working through you. You cannot manifest this level of understanding without concepts, lots of study, and lots of hard work. Although it can be shaped by concepts and training, ultimately this kind of knowing does not come from concepts alone. It is not the kind of know-how that you can easily capture in reflective thought. It is a wide-ranging set of practical skills that knows by doing. Often it is best expressed in the language of poetry.

To one degree or another, most manual therapists have experienced this kind of inspired freedom when working with a client. Typically, especially in the beginning stages of our career, it shows up in our sessions now and then in varying degrees of intensity and depth. But, if we really want to explore the contours of getting manual therapy, we need to explore it where it most clearly manifests—in those all-encompassing, creative moments when your work becomes more like an inspired performance of a piece of music than just the application of technique or following a protocol. During such grand moments, your grasp of the work unfolds with an uncanny clarity of intent that makes your every intervention effortlessly achieve its greatest effect, often leaving you breathless.*

Before we look at an example of "getting it," let me remind you that we are looking at the extreme all-out manifestations of inspired work, because it promises to reveal more clearly the contours of this experience. These wonderful moments of inspired work come and go. They vary greatly in their intensity in our day-to-day practice, whether you have been a manual therapist for thirty years or thirty days. I am using these extreme examples to make a point. I am not suggesting that you are doing good work only when your sessions exemplify the all-out extremes discussed here.

Martial artist Peter Ralston relates an incident that illustrates an aspect of what happens when you get it. When he was a student of judo, he wanted to practice more hours than his dojo was open. He solved this problem when he stumbled upon the idea of practicing his throws in his mind. While practicing in his mind and on the mat he discovered something amazing. "While sitting there one evening working on the throws in my mind, in a flash I simply "got" judo. I got what it *was* . . . I understood

---

*For a much more detailed description of how the transformative turn to a creative performance occurs and is experienced, see Chapter Four in my book *Spacious Body* (Berkeley: North Atlantic Books, 1995).

what the founder of judo, Jigoro Kano, had in mind. Judo was supposed to be easy! Suddenly, I didn't have to learn technique after technique searching for 'judo'—I could create techniques from my new understanding. It seemed unbelievable, even after my success with mind training, but the power of this insight was proven by an immediate change in my abilities. Overnight, I became good at judo."[52] He practiced visualization and actual judo diligently and constantly until he suddenly got it. At the very same moment he got judo his abilities were instantly enhanced, and he became the living, breathing manifestation of judo. He was able to drop his thinking self and surrender to the intelligence of his sentient body.

Suddenly, he was not just someone who practiced and understood judo; he was the embodiment of judo itself. Notice that he said he did not have to learn technique after technique in search of judo. Because he got judo, he was able to discover creative new techniques from his new bodily understanding and perception that were precisely designed to deal with the present situation. Creating new techniques was possible because of his shift to a practical, whole-body understanding of judo.

Similarly, manual therapists who get it, find that exploring holistic seeing yields creative ways of working that are not dependent upon formulistic protocols. From their new understanding, they create new techniques, new ways of seeing, new ways of manipulating, and a seemingly endless number of varied and sundry ways to intervene. All the while, their sessions become more and more geared to the individual needs of the clients and less and less about being true to external standards and protocols. When therapists get it, their sessions do not get sidetracked by their unsettled, self-critical, thinking mind.

They become better manual therapists. Their hands-on skills and perceptual vitality are both enhanced. They are no longer bound by recipes, often get better change with less effort, see more clearly and holistically where their clients' patterns of strain are, and create new techniques in response to their clients' needs. Surprisingly, even if they employ the very same techniques and treatment strategies they have always employed, they get better results.

Getting it is not a one-time thing. Getting it implies you have to be seized with this kind of understanding, not just once, but over and over again as you develop and evolve throughout your career. Then you become the living, breathing manifestation of manual skills and the skillful seeing that comes with it.

For an even richer understanding of getting it, we turn next to the great Taoist philosopher, Chuang Tzu. What follows is a respectful, but slightly altered version of Chuang Tzu's "Cutting Up an Ox." The version of "Cutting Up an Ox" from which I created "The Tao of Rolfing SI" comes from Thomas Merton's *The Way of Chuang Tzu*.[53] The original story is about a Taoist butcher. I changed the text in a few critical places—surprisingly few, when you think about it—in order to make it about a Taoist Rolfer. This story first appeared under the title of "The Tao of Rolfing SI."[54]

THE TAO OF ROLFING SI

John's Rolfer was demonstrating
His art on a volunteer from the audience.
Out went a hand,
Down went a shoulder,
He planted a foot,
His fingers joined with the flesh,
The volunteer's body shuddered,
Softened, lengthened,
And suddenly it was integrated and at ease.
With a whisper,
His fingers pulsated with the flesh,
It's like a gentle breeze.
Rhythm! Timing!
Like a sacred dance,
Like "The Mulberry grove,"
Like ancient harmonies!

"Good work!" John exclaimed.
"Your method is faultless!"
"Method?" said the Rolfer,
His hands still in contact with the volunteer,
"What I follow is the Tao of Rolfing SI,
Beyond all methods!

"When I first began to
Rolf, I would see before me
The whole body
All in one mass.
After three years,
I no longer saw this mass.
I made distinctions among parts.
But now, I see nothing
With the eye. My whole being
Apprehends.
My senses are idle. The spirit,
Free to work without the recipe,
Follows its own instinct
Guided by the natural Palintonic lines,
By the secret opening, the hidden space,
My hands find their own way.
I use no excessive force, I scour no bones.

A good bodyworker needs a vacation
once a year; he works with great effort
And large calluses.
A poor bodyworker needs a vacation
Every month—he mashes fascia with sweating,
Swollen hands.

I am not a bodyworker,
And I have Rolfed this way for 19 years.
My hands have touched
Thousands of people.
Yet they are soft and supple
Like a baby's.
Never do I feel pain or dis-ease.

There are spaces in the body,
My fingers can be either fat or lean:
When this deftness
Finds that space,
There is all the room you need!
It goes like a breeze!
Hence I have Rolfed this way for 19 years
Free of calluses and all effort.

"True, there is sometimes
Tough tissue. I feel it coming,
I slow down, I watch closely,
Hold back, barely move my hands,
And whoosh! Something opens and makes way

Gently flowing like a river.
"Then I withdraw my hands,
I stand still
And let the joy of my work
Sink in. I wash my hands
And my work is done."

John said "This is it.
My Rolfer has shown me
How I ought to live
My own life!"

Chuang Tzu's story is a wonderful description of a practitioner who gets it with his whole being and, by example, demonstrates ". . . how I ought to live my own life." In it, we see similarities to Ralston's account and the experiences of running down a mountain and walking meditation. For the most part, the experience of getting it with your whole being is the same whether we are talking about getting manual therapy, judo, cutting up an ox, walking meditation, or performing a piece of music. Because goals and procedures by which the goals are reached for each activity are different, how they are performed obviously will not be the same. But the experience of effortless freedom is common to all forms of inspiration.

Similar to Ralston's experience, the Taoist Rolfer was able to work impeccably and creatively with what each individual's unique structure required without being constrained by formulistic protocols or having to deal with the interference of his thinking self. He was able to work this way because it completely and fully flowed from his living his practice. Because he was free enough to become one with his client, his hands became deft at finding and creating space and allowing tough tissue to release itself without effort.

He no longer perceives the body as an assembly of parts. He instinctively perceives holistically. He now sees symptoms as modifications of larger patterns and primary strain patterns as relational imbalanced wholes. Whereas he used to work with direct muscular effort and will, he now works effortlessly with his whole body and finds that his hands are capable of allowing a space for the kind of change the body can afford. As a result, order naturally and necessarily appears. Before he even places his hands on his client, because of his new orientation, his very presence is often enough to initiate change. By pre-reflectively accessing the reservoir of bodily know-how, he feels as if something is working through him and making room for change. He has become like the poet whose poems write themselves.

Most intriguing of all is an experience he reports on that Ralston overlooked in his account: an enhanced perceptual ability that both includes and goes beyond the five senses. The Taoist Rolfer says that when he first began to work, he saw the whole body all in one mass. Then after three years he no longer saw the mass. Instead, he saw distinctions and parts. Even though the perceptual vitality of all his senses is greatly enhanced, now he sees nothing with the eye because his whole being apprehends. He discovered what many practitioners discover after years of devoting themselves to their art—his whole being is the sensorium. Not only can he perceive more holistically and work with more clarity and precision, his ability to perceive goes beyond the five senses, and he finds himself able to perceive with his body and energy. As a result, he can work effectively on the many levels of order-thwarters that are delineated by the categories of assessment in Chapter Two. With unerring precision, his sentient body often knows where and how to work on his client, even before he ever brings it into reflective awareness.

Sentient Body Know-How

Getting manual therapy puts you in touch with a reservoir of bodily know-how. As a way to catch a glimpse of this kind of freedom in action, imagine what it might be like to engage in a match after getting judo. For the duration of the match, you would not be thinking about how to move or counter your opponent's move. Instead, you would find yourself moving effortlessly with complete freedom, making all the right choices without breaking the flow of one movement into the next by means of too much planning or thinking. The same goes for an inspired manual therapist, an inspired musician, or an inspired butcher. Their every movement occurs where the intention to move and the actual movement are experienced as one and the same action.

This free flow of one movement into the next is not a matter of your planning what to do, willing your body to move, and then moving it, as we saw in Chapter Eleven. Rather, during the judo match, there is only just effortless, pre-reflectively conscious, intelligent, purposeful throwing of your opponent and countering his or her moves. Later when you report on what you were pre-reflectively doing, you bring it into reflective awareness and think about it. But the minute you think about it, the exquisite free flow of one movement into the next disappears.

Whether we are considering judo throws, manual therapy, or playing a musical instrument, this intelligent and effortless freedom of moving and acting only happens when we are not attending to what we are doing. Under these conditions, there is no reflective intention in play and no thinking self to get in the way. Unless you are learning some new throws or struggling to move after an injury, you do not typically move by reflectively intending to move and then moving. If you are a master of judo, in the heat of a match where each movement freely flows into the next, your every move would be a manifestation of a pre-reflective understanding of the being of judo. Your actions are the discourse of getting it and the language of the being of judo is found in how you move. If you want to know whether someone gets the being of a practice and speaks its language, watch him or her move.

If your opponent also got judo, the least bit of thinking about your actions could be your downfall. If you did attend to what you were doing, a gap would appear in your freely flowing movement and in an instant your opponent would immediately sense your vulnerability. Just as quickly, your opponent would slam you to the mat and you would surely lose.

Similarly, a seasoned manual therapist knows how to get out of the way by dropping his or her reflective self and letting the pre-reflective bodily know-how reveal what needs to be done and then performing the appropriate manipulations. Effortlessly, from his or her whole body understanding, one manipulation freely flows into the next—intelligently, yet without the compulsion to reflect on what he or she is doing or without the need to grasp his or her actions in representational thinking.

Conclusion

The fact that the Western world has stood in denial of the body for over 2,500 years makes it difficult for many to understand the intelligence of the sentient body, that some aspect of consciousness is a somatic event.

When you add to these inherited blinders the fact that we are also not very cognizant of how much of our daily experience takes place at the pre-reflective level of consciousness, where this kind of bodily know-how is always operating, it is easy to see why it is so difficult for us to grasp this kind of bodily intelligence. After all, how do you grasp something that only appears when you are not thinking about it? The minute we try to think about or reflect on it, it ceases being a freely flowing activity we are pre-reflectively living through and becomes an object of thought.

Given that we tend to be more comfortable as detached, spectatorial percipients who reduce all thinking to the reflective level of thought and shun the rest as mere idiosyncratic subjectivity, given that we cannot grasp or represent to ourselves much of this sentient whole-body knowing in reflective thought, and given that we do not trust what we cannot experience in reflection, it is no wonder we remain skeptical, confused, or unsure about our experience. But when you finally surrender to the way of knowing that comes with getting it, you learn to trust your sentient body's intelligence, and your work becomes effortless and inspired.

After making our way through the theory and practice of manual therapy to our present understanding, we come to a rather interesting conclusion. Whether we look at the experience of creating art, appreciating art, tromping in the snow, performing art, receiving manual therapy, performing manual therapy, walking meditation, experiencing the tunnel of light, or just being here, we are looking at different depths of the same experience of coming home. Each appears to be a different portal from the others because each takes a somewhat different path in finding its way home. When it is at its very best, manual therapy is a portal that can help clients arrive at the same experience—the performance and realization of human freedom. The way freedom is realized for the client and the way it is experienced by the therapist are different paths to the same experience of coming home.

NOTES

Chapter One: Homecoming, Part I

1. Samuel Todes, *Body and World* (Cambridge, MA: MIT Press, 2001).
2. Ibid., 176.
3. Ida P. Rolf, *Rolfing: The Integration of Human Structure* (Santa Monica: Harper & Row, 1977), 31.
4. Ida P. Rolf, *Ida Rolf Talks about Rolfing and Physical Reality* (New York: Harper & Row, 1978), 189.

Chapter Two: The Territory

5. Harold Roth, *Original Tao* (New York: Columbia University Press, 1999), 104.
6. John Cage, *Silence* (Cambridge, MA: MIT Press, 1966), 16.

Chapter Three: In Search of Principles

7. Philip E. Greenman, *Principles of Manual Medicine* (Baltimore: Williams and Wilkins, 1989), 182.
8. R. C. Schafer and L. J. Faye, *Motion Palpation and Chiropractic Technique— Principles of Dynamic Chiropractic* (Huntington Beach: The Motion Palpation Institute, 1990), 33.
9. Ron Kurtz, *Body-Centered Psychotherapy: The Hakomi Method* (Mendocino: LifeRhythm, 1990), 29.
10. Robert C. Ward, "Myofascial Release Concepts," in *Rational Manual Therapies* (Baltimore: Williams and Wilkins, 1993), 237.
11. Fred L. Mitchell Jr., "Elements of Muscle Energy Technique," in *Rational Manual Therapies* (Baltimore: Williams and Wilkins, 1993), 285.
12. G. D. Maitland, *Vertebral Manipulation* (Boston: Butterworth-Heinemann Ltd, 1986), 3.
13. G. D. Maitland, *Peripheral Manipulation* (Boston: Butterworth-Heinemann Ltd, 1991), 1.

14. Alan J. Grodin and Robert I. Cantu, "Soft Tissue Mobilization," in *Rational Manual Therapies* (Baltimore: Williams and Wilkins, 1993), 218.

15. Michael L. Kuchera, "Gravitational Stress, Musculoligamentous Strain, and Postural Alignment," in *SPINE: State of the Art Reviews* 9, no. 2 (May 1995), 463–490.

Chapter Four: The Principles of Intervention

16. Maurice Merleau-Ponty, *The Structure of Behavior* (Boston: Beacon Press, 1963), 131.

Chapter Six: Seeing

17. Henri Bortoft, *Taking Appearances Seriously: The Dynamic Way of Seeing in Goethe and European Thought* (Edinburgh: Floris Books, 2012), 46.

18. Henri Bortoft, *The Wholeness of Nature: Goethe's Way toward a Science of Conscious Participation in Nature* (New York: Lindisfarna Press, 1996), 281.

19. Ibid., 50.

20. Calvin O. Schrag, *Existence and Being* (Evanston: Northwestern University Press, 1969), 82.

21. Martin Heidegger, *Being and Time*, trans. Joan Stambaugh (New York: State University of New York Press, 1996), 30.

22. Bortoft, *Taking Appearances Seriously*, 49.

23. Ibid., 25.

Chapter Seven: The Beauty of Normality

24. Ida P. Rolf, *Ida Rolf Talks about Rolfing and Physical Reality* (New York: Harper and Row, 1978), 186.

25. Ibid., 180.

26. Ibid., 96.

27. Ibid., 201.

28. John Cottingham, S. W. Porges, and K. Richmond, "Shifts in Pelvic Inclination Angle and Parasympathetic Tone Produced by Rolfing Soft Tissue Manipulation," *Physical Therapy* 68, no. 9 (1988): 1364–1370.

29. John Cottingham, S. W. Porges, and T. Lyon, "Effects of Soft Tissue Mobilization (Rolfing Pelvic Left) on Parasympathetic Tone in Two Age Groups," *Physical Therapy* 68, no. 3 (1988): 352–356.

30. John Cottingham and Jeffrey Maitland, "A Three-Paradigm Treatment Model Using Soft Tissue Mobilization and Guided Movement—Awareness Techniques for Patients with Chronic Low Back Pain: A Case Study," *The Journal of Orthopedic and Sports Physical Therapy* 26, no. 3 (1997): 155–167.

31. John Cottingham and Jeffrey Maitland, "Integrating Manual and Movement Therapy with Philosophical Counseling for Treatment of a Patient with ALS: A Case Study That Explores the Principles of Holistic Intervention," *Alternative Therapies in Health and Medicine* 6, no. 2 (2000): 128, 120–127.

32. Ibid., 189.

33. Ibid., 69.

34. Henri Bortoft, *The Wholeness of Nature: Goethe's Way toward a Science of Conscious Participation in Nature* (Edinburgh: Lindisfarna Press, 1996), 55.

35. Ibid., 281.

36. Frederick Amrine, "The Metamorphosis of the Scientist," in *Goethe's Way of Science* (New York: State University of New York Press, 1998).

37. Ida P. Rolf, *Rolfing: The Integration of Human Structure* (Santa Monica: Harper & Row, 1977), 65.

Chapter Eight: Sentient Body

38. Maurice Merleau-Ponty, *The Structure of Behavior* (Boston: Beacon Press, 1963), 131.

39. Henri Bortoft, *The Wholeness of Nature: Goethe's Way toward a Science of Conscious Participation in Nature* (New York: Lindisfarna Press, 1996), 1–23.

40. Mae-Wan Ho, *The Rainbow and the Worm: The Physics of Organisms*, 2nd ed. (Hackensack: World Scientific Publishing Co., 1998).

41. Gregory Bateson, *Mind and Nature: A Necessary Unity* (New York: Hampton Press, 1979), 101.

42. Daniel Dennett, *Darwin's Dangerous Idea* (New York: Simon and Schuster, 1995), 300.

43. Daniel Dennett, *Kinds of Minds: Toward an Understanding of Consciousness* (New York: Basic Books, 1996).

44. David Chalmers, "Facing Up to the Hard Problem of Consciousness," *Journal of Consciousness Studies* 2 (1995): 200–219.

45. Frank Jackson, "Epiphenomenal Qualia," *Philosophical Quarterly* 32 (1982): 127–136.

Chapter Nine: Appropriating Gravity

46. Ida P. Rolf, *Rolfing: The Integration of Human Structures* (New York: Harper & Row, 1971), 65.
47. Ibid., 33.
48. Ibid., 34.

Chapter Ten: In Praise of Subjectivity

49. M. C. Dillon, *Merleau-Ponty's Ontology* (Evanston: Northwestern University Press, 1988), 110–111.

Chapter Eleven: Homecoming, Part II: Where You Always and Already Are

50. Thomas W. Myers, *Anatomy Trains: Myofascial Meridians for Manual and Movement Therapists*, 3rd ed. (New York: Churchill Livingstone, 2014), 31.
51. Jeffrey Maitland, *Spacious Body* (Berkeley: North Atlantic Books, 1995), 63.

Chapter Twelve: The Poetics of Manual Therapy

52. Peter Ralston, *Zen Body-Being* (Berkeley: North Atlantic Books, 2006), 16–17.
53. Thomas Merton, *The Way of Chuang Tzu* (New York: New Directions, 1995).
54. Jeffrey Maitland, "The Tao of Rolfing S1," *Rolf Lines* 18, no. 3 (May/June 1990), 1.

RELEVANT CITATIONS

The ideas that inform the writing of this book have evolved and developed from two practices. One is the practice of Zen. The other is the practice of contemplating philosophically the practice and teaching of Rolfing SI. In a very real sense my Rolfing practice and my Rolfing classes are my laboratory. Today, I find myself in the agreeable position of being able to engage in my love of philosophy by philosophically contemplating my love of Rolfing while bringing benefit to others.

I originally decided to chronicle my discoveries in the form of articles. I had no intention of writing another book. But as more articles appeared I began to see the emergence of a book. Below is a list of articles that contributed in one form or another to articulating the orientation that finally grew into this book.

"Orthotropism and the Unbinding of Morphological Potential." *Rolf Lines* 29, issue 1 (2001): 15–24.

"Patterns That Perpetuate Themselves." *Journal of Structural Integration* 37, issue 3 (2009): 23–30.

"Moving toward Our Evolutionary Potential." *Rolf Lines* XXIV, no. 2 (May 1996): 5–23.

"Radical Somatics and Philosophical Counseling." *Rolf Lines* XXVII, no. 2 (Spring 1999): 29–40.

"Perception and the Cognitive Theory of Life: Or How Did Matter Become Conscious of Itself?" *Rolf Lines* XXVII, no. 4 (Fall 1999): 5–13.

"Seeing." *Structural Integration: Journal of the Rolf Institute* 42, no. 2 (December 2014).

BIBLIOGRAPHY

Amrine, Frederick. "The Metamorphosis of the Scientist." In *Goethe's Way of Science*. New York: State University of New York Press, 1998.

Bateson, Gregory. *Mind and Nature: A Necessary Unity*. New York: Hampton Press, 1979.

Bortoft, Henri. *The Wholeness of Nature: Goethe's Way toward a Science of Conscious Participation in Nature*. New York: Lindisfarna Press, 1996.

Bortoft, Henri. *Taking Appearances Seriously: The Dynamic Way of Seeing in Goethe and European Thought*. Edinburgh: Floris Books, 2012.

Cage, John. *Silence*. Cambridge, MA: MIT Press, 1966.

Chadwick, Ruth, ed. *Immanuel Kant: Critical Assessments*. Routledge, 1992.

Chalmers, David. "Facing Up to the Hard Problem of Consciousness." *Journal of Consciousness Studies* 2 (1995): 200–219.

Cottingham, John, and Jeffrey Maitland. "A Three-Paradigm Treatment Model Using Soft Tissue Mobilization and Guided Movement—Awareness Techniques for a Patient with Chronic Low Back Pain: A Case Study." *Journal of Orthopedic and Sports Physical Therapy* 26, no. 3 (1997): 155–167.

Cottingham, John, and Jeffrey Maitland. "Integrating Manual and Movement Therapy with Philosophical Counseling for Treatment of a Patient with Amyotrophic Lateral Sclerosis: A Case Study That Explores the Principles of Holistic Intervention." *Alternative Therapies in Health and Medicine* 6, no. 2 (2000): 120–127.

Cottingham, John, S. W. Porges, and K. Richmond. "Shifts in Pelvic Inclination Angle and Parasympathetic Tone Produced by Rolfing Soft Tissue Manipulation." *Physical Therapy* 68, no. 9 (1988): 1364–1370.

Cottingham, John, S. W. Porges, and T. Lyon. "Effects of Soft Tissue Mobilization (Rolfing Pelvic Left) on Parasympathetic Tone in Two Age Groups." *Physical Therapy* 68, no. 3 (1988): 352–356.

Dennett, Daniel. *Darwin's Dangerous Idea*. New York: Simon and Schuster, 1995.

Dennett, Daniel. *Kinds of Minds: Toward an Understanding of Consciousness*. New York: Basic Books, 1996.

Dillon, M.C. *Merleau-Ponty's Ontology.* Evanston: Northwestern University Press, 1988.

Fisher, John, and Jeffrey Maitland. "The Subjectivist Turn in Aesthetics: A Critical Analysis of Kant's Theory of Appreciation." *The Review of Metaphysics* 27, no. 4 (1974): 726–751.

Greenman, Philip E. *Principles of Manual Medicine.* Baltimore: Williams and Wilkins, 1989.

Grodin, Alan J., and Robert I. Cantu. "Soft Tissue Mobilization." In *Rational Manual Therapies*, 218. Baltimore: Williams and Wilkins, 1993.

Heidegger, Martin. *Being and Time.* Translated by Joan Stambaugh. New York: State University of New York Press, 1996.

Ho, Mae-Wan. *The Rainbow and the Worm: The Physics of Organisms.* 2nd ed. Hackensack: World Scientific Publishing Co., 1998.

Jackson, Frank. "Epiphenomenal Qualia." *Philosophical Quarterly* 32 (1982): 127–136.

Kendall, Florence P., Elizabeth K. McCreary, Patricia G. Provance, Mary M. Rodgers, and William A. Romani. *Muscles: Testing and Function.* 3rd ed. Baltimore: Williams and Wilkins, 1983.

Kuchera, Michael L. "Gravitational Stress, Musculoligamentous Strain, and Postural Alignment." In *SPINE: State of the Art Reviews* 9, no. 2 (May 1995): 463–490.

Kurtz, Ron. *Body-Centered Psychotherapy: The Hakomi Method.* Mendocino: LifeRhythm, 1990.

Maitland, G. D. *Vertebral Manipulation.* Boston: Butterworth-Heinemann Ltd, 1986.

Maitland, G. D. *Peripheral Manipulation.* Boston: Butterworth-Heinemann Ltd, 1991.

Maitland, Jeffrey. "An Ontology of Appreciation: Kant's Aesthetics and the Problem of Metaphysics." *Journal of the British Society for Phenomenology* 13, no. 1 (January 1982): 45–68.

Maitland, Jeffrey. "The Tao of Rolfing SI." *Rolf Lines* 18, no. 3 (May/June 1990).

Maitland, Jeffrey. *Spacious Body: Explorations in Somatic Ontology.* Berkeley: North Atlantic Books, 1995.

Maitland, Jeffrey. "Moving toward Our Evolutionary Potential." *Rolf Lines* XXIV, no. 2 (May 1996): 5–23.

Maitland, Jeffrey. "Radical Somatics and Philosophical Counseling." *Rolf Lines* XXVII, no. 2 (Spring 1999), 29–40.

Maitland, Jeffrey. "Perception and the Cognitive Theory of Life: Or How Did Matter Become Conscious of Itself?" *Rolf Lines* XXVII, no. 4 (Fall 1999): 5–13.

Maitland, Jeffrey. "Orthotropism and the Unbinding of Morphological Potential." *Rolf Lines* 29, issue 1 (2001): 15–24.

Maitland, Jeffrey. "Patterns That Perpetuate Themselves." *Journal of Structural Integration* 37, issue 3 (2009): 23–30.

Maitland, Jeffrey. *Mind Body Zen*. Berkeley: North Atlantic Books, 2010.

Merleau-Ponty, Maurice. *The Structure of Behavior*. Boston: Beacon Press, 1963.

Merton, Thomas. *The Way of Chuang Tzu*. New York: New Directions, 1995.

Mitchell Jr., Fred L. "Elements of Muscle Energy Technique." In *Rational Manual Therapies*, 285. Baltimore: Williams and Wilkins, 1993.

Myers, Thomas W. *Anatomy Trains: Myofascial Meridians for Manual and Movement Therapists*. 3rd ed. New York: Churchill Livingstone, 2012.

Oschman, James L. *Energy Medicine: The Scientific Basis*. Edinburgh: Churchill Livingston, 2000.

Oschman, James L. *Energy Medicine in Therapeutics and Human Performance*. Philadelphia: Butterworth Heinmann, 2003.

Ralston, Peter. *Zen Body-Being*. Berkeley: North Atlantic Books, 2006.

Rolf, Ida P. *Rolfing: The Integration of Human Structure*. Santa Monica: Harper & Row, 1977.

Rolf, Ida P. *Ida Rolf Talks about Rolfing and Physical Reality*. New York: Harper & Row, 1978.

Roth, Harold. *Original Tao*. New York: Columbia University Press, 1999.

Schafer, R. C., and L. J. Faye. *Motion Palpation and Chiropractic Technique— Principles of Dynamic Chiropractic*. Huntington Beach: The Motion Palpation Institute, 1990.

Schrag, Calvin O. *Existence Being*. Evanston: Northwestern University Press, 1969.

Sills, Franklyn. *Craniosacral Biodynamics*. Vol. 2, The Primal Midline and the Organization of the Body. Berkeley: North Atlantic Books, 2003.

Todes, Samuel. *Body and World*. Cambridge, MA: MIT Press, 2001.

Ward, Robert C. "Myofascial Release Concepts." In *Rational Manual Therapies*, 237. Baltimore: Williams and Wilkins, 1993.

ACKNOWLEDGMENTS

As an ordained Zen monk, advanced Rolfer and Rolfing Instructor, and former professor of philosophy, I stand at the confluence of three great rivers of thought. When I finally learned to not insist on my way and truly listen, this confluence afforded me insight and knowledge. I have gained so much that I could never begin to sort out where it all came from. In truth, these insights came from everywhere: the wind in the trees, dark recesses of the brain, the turn of a phrase, watching a client shed years of debilitating pain, appreciating the beauty of integrated movement that appears with attaining the freedom of embodiment, the support and love of my family.... and, of course, what I learned from my teachers, students, and clients. Any attempt to acknowledge all the influences and support I have received over the years is probably impossible. My gratitude extends to all the unseen forces and people who made this project possible.

I deeply appreciate the training I received in Rolfing SI at the Rolf Institute of Structural Integration. I benefited greatly from studying and teaching with Jan Sultan, a truly gifted teacher. From him I learned the most about how to teach Rolfing SI. I was privileged to also teach with and learn from Senior Rolfing Instructor, Michael Salveson, also a creative master of the art. I am grateful to have studied with two other recognized masters of the art, Emmett Hutchins and Peter Melchior. All four of these teachers manifested an indefatigable commitment and an uncanny ability to impart Rolf's vision. I am a much better Rolfer and Rolfing Instructor because of their influence. I also had the privilege of teaching a number of Advanced Rolfing classes with Peter Schwind, a gifted Rolfer in his own right. With great fondness I recall the many evenings we conversed about a wide range of topics, from the philosophy and practice of manual therapy to the medicinal properties of wine. Special thanks are due to Ray McCall, Advanced Rolfer and Rolfing Instructor, for his creative collaboration in designing our first workshop in *seeing*. His practiced and sensitive eye was invaluable to the project. Many thanks to the practitioners whose openhearted participation contributed to the success of this first-of-a-kind experimental workshop in perception.

Once more I wish to express my gratitude to my colleague and mentor, Calvin O. Schrag. Even though he is a philosopher, not a manual therapist, I could not have written this book without his far-reaching and learned influence.

I also must also acknowledge my friend and colleague, Rihab Yaqub. Her keen eye when coupled with her forthright unabashed commentary was enormously helpful to me. Coming from a similar clarity of purpose and critical insight, my friend Christina Burawa helped steer me away from flights of philosophical fancy. I also want to express my appreciation of Anne Hoff's expert and conscientious work as editor in chief of *Structural Integration: The Journal of the Rolf Institute* and Deanna Melnychuk's careful editing of my manuscripts.

Also, I am very fortunate to have as my family doctor Bradley Williams, MD. Part shaman, part metaphysician, part soothsayer, part priest, part psychologist, and altogether human—he truly deserves the title of physician. I have learned much from him and have benefited greatly from his work.

I would be truly remiss if I did not acknowledge the profound influence of my Zen teacher. Even as he received manual therapy from me, he continued to wordlessly teach me.

Many thanks are due my publisher Richard Grossinger of North Atlantic Books. His vision saw a place for my work and Tim McKee, Hisae Matsuda, Amy Reff, Jasmine Hromjak, and Brad Greene made it possible to effortlessly bring forth my book to press.

Finally, I want to acknowledge the unflagging support of a dear departed friend. He always had my back and life has been better from having known him. Thank you, Sokai.

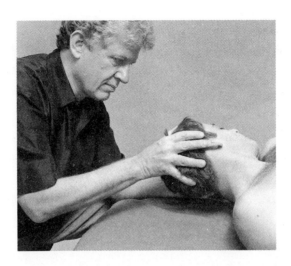

ABOUT THE AUTHOR

JEFFREY MAITLAND, PhD, has spent most of his adult life deeply investigating Zen practice, philosophy, and the nature of healing. He is a Zen monk ordained by Joshu Sasaki Roshi, an energy healer, a Certified Advanced Rolfer, a former professor of philosophy at Purdue University, and a philosophical counselor. With thirty-plus years of experience and over 5,000 hours of training, Dr. Maitland is one of seven Advanced Rolfing Instructors in the world. He employs a gentle, non-formulistic approach to Rolfing and is highly skilled in visceral manipulation, biodynamic craniosacral, energetic, and cold laser therapy. Internationally known as an author, instructor, innovator, and expert in soft tissue manipulation, his advice is often sought by other professionals. Maitland teaches workshops and classes in myofascial manipulation to physical therapists and other health care professionals. Maitland has published and presented many papers on the theory of somatic manual therapy, Zen, philosophy, and Rolfing. His research, articles, and book reviews are published in numerous professional journals.